W9-CHZ-406

HELP WANTED: CAREGIVER

A GUIDE TO HELPING YOUR LOVED ONE COPE WITH SERIOUS ILLNESS

BY LAURA J. PINCHOT

Hygeia Media
An imprint of the Oncology Nursing Society
Pittsburgh, Pennsylvania

ONS Publishing Division
Publisher: Leonard Mafrica, MBA, CAE
Director of Publications: Barbara Sigler, RN, MNEd
Managing Editor: Lisa M. George, BA
Technical Content Editor: Angela D. Klimaszewski, RN, MSN
Staff Editor: Amy Nicoletti, BA
Graphic Designer: Dany Sjoen

Library of Congress Cataloging-in-Publication Data
Pinchot, Laura J.
Help wanted, caregiver : a guide to helping your loved one cope with serious illness / By Laura J. Pinchot.
p. cm.
ISBN 978-1-890504-97-7
1. Caregivers. 2. Critically ill--Home care. I. Title.
RA645.3.P56 2011
362'.0425--dc22

2010024957

Publisher's Note
This book is published by the Oncology Nursing Society (ONS). ONS neither represents nor guarantees that the practices described herein will, if followed, ensure safe and effective patient care. The recommendations contained in this book reflect ONS's judgment regarding the state of general knowledge and practice in the field as of the date of publication. The recommendations may not be appropriate for use in all circumstances. Those who use this book should make their own determinations regarding specific safe and appropriate patient-care practices, taking into account the personnel, equipment, and practices available at the hospital or other facility at which they are located. The author and publisher cannot be held responsible for any liability incurred as a consequence from the use or application of any of the contents of this book. Figures and tables are used as examples only. They are not meant to be all-inclusive, nor do they represent endorsement of any particular institution by ONS. Mention of specific products and opinions related to those products do not indicate or imply endorsement by ONS. Web sites mentioned are provided for information only; the hosts are responsible for their own content and availability. Unless otherwise indicated, dollar amounts reflect U.S. dollars.

ONS publications are originally published in English. Publishers wishing to translate ONS publications must contact the ONS Publishing Division about licensing arrangements. ONS publications cannot be translated without obtaining written permission from ONS. (Individual tables and figures that are reprinted or adapted require additional permission from the original source.) Because translations from English may not always be accurate or precise, ONS disclaims any responsibility for inaccuracies in words or meaning that may occur as a result of the translation. Readers relying on precise information should check the original English version.

Printed in the United States of America

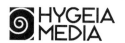

An imprint of the Oncology Nursing Society

This book was inspired by very special people who exemplify quintessential caregivers: Bob and Romaine Evans, Harry and Linda Davis, Lisa and Robert McCarl, the Pinchot family, Lois McCarl, Sharon McCarl, Jeff and Debbie Baird, Dr. Rebecca Cox-Davenport, and Suzanne Kovel.

TABLE OF CONTENTS

FOREWORD

Help Wanted: Caregiver is an invaluable resource for all who find themselves in the position of caring for a loved one who cannot completely care for himself. The book redefines present-day caregivers as care coordinators, and that's an important distinction to make because it implies that caring for a sick parent, child, or sibling is not a task any of us should undertake alone.

The challenge, though, is where to find help, and this book makes it easy while framing the discussion in terms of finding a new way to look at an often hopeless-feeling situation: "A primary family caregiver's job is big essentially because this person is performing the basic activities of two people. . . . It is natural to feel overwhelmed, but this is not an unmanageable situation. Sometimes perspective just needs adjustment."

This handbook is short and clear enough that reading the whole thing will not feel burdensome, but individuals can also pick the chapters best suited to their own questions. There are chapters both on homecare and institutional options, which outline the benefits of both situations and discuss which types of patients are best suited to these different care environments. In later chapters, frank discussions of how to obtain financial assistance, when to establish a power of attorney, and the importance of caregivers making time for their own lives portray caring for someone as achievable without the caregiver having to file for bankruptcy or putting her own needs indefinitely on hold.

The sixth and final chapter, "Help Wanted: Family Counselor," talks honestly about how emotionally taxing it can be to provide care for another and encourages strong communication skills as a way of keeping the situation from wearing you down emotionally. Chapter sections subtitled "Listen," "Choose Your Words Wisely," and "Take a Walk in Their Shoes" all encourage empathy for the person needing care while also acknowledging that maintaining empathy is hard work.

Finally, the appendices are full of common-sense tips and lists of resources that should be considered in the whirl of caregiving responsibilities. Advice such as "Learn CPR," and "Assemble a first aid kit" is invaluable because it focuses attention on the fact that the caregiver is needed for an ill person who can no longer safely take care of herself. The list of Internet resources is thorough without being overwhelming and thus is extremely helpful.

Americans are living longer and longer, and advances in medicine mean that ill or disabled individuals are surviving injuries and illnesses that a decade ago might have claimed their lives. These accomplishments of medical science are of course wonderful, but at the same time they mean that more and more of us will, at some point in our lives, become caregivers. When that difficult but important task falls to me I will, with gratitude and relief, reach for *Help Wanted: Caregiver*.

Theresa Brown, RN

Theresa Brown, RN, is an oncology nurse, the author of *Critical Care: A New Nurse Faces Death, Life, and Everything in Between*, and a regular contributor to the *New York Times* blog "Well."

ACKNOWLEDGMENTS

I would like to extend a special thank you to my mentors, colleagues, family, and dear friends, who provided invaluable guidance and support throughout the writing process.

CHAPTER 1

INTRODUCTION

Compassion is the hallmark of human beings. No other species on the planet cares for their sick, aged, or young to the extent that we do. Throughout the natural cycle of health, illness, and aging, each of us will likely be in the position that we will need to rely on the compassion of people beyond the medical community and social services—caregivers—to assist us as we cope with a temporary illness or injury, permanent disability, or declining health. More than 50 million people in the United States provide care for a family member, friend, or neighbor who is chronically ill or disabled (National Family Caregivers Association [NFCA], 2000, n.d.; U.S. Department of Health and Human Services [DHHS], 1998). Surveys have shown informal family caregivers range in age from as young as 8 years old to older than 65 (DHHS, 1998; NFCA, 2000, n.d.). Most of us will be called upon to fulfill the role of caregiver at some point in our lives, some of us multiple times. Former First Lady and caregiver advocate Rosalynn Carter efficiently summed up who will fill this role: "One of my colleagues once said, 'There are only four kinds of people in the world—those who have been caregivers, those who currently are caregivers, those who will be caregivers, and those who need caregivers'" (McLeod, 2003, p. 5).

Who Needs Caregivers?

- Children and adults with disabilities, including intellectual, physical, and emotional disabilities
- Older adults who need help with daily activities or who can no longer take care of themselves
- People recovering from major surgery
- Individuals with a long-term illness, such as cancer or multiple sclerosis
- People recovering from a serious injury
- Veterans who are returning from active duty with serious trauma, dismemberment, or post-traumatic stress disorder

The term *caregiver* can be used generally to describe people who assist others with tasks of daily life and oversee and protect those who may not be able to watch out for themselves. It also describes those who provide basic medical assistance, such as ensuring that medication is taken as prescribed or helping with physical therapy exercises. However, for purposes of this book, the term will be used to describe informal caregivers who are not paid to provide these types of services, such as family members, friends, or neighbors.

Who Can Be a Family Caregiver?

• Spouse/partner	• Other relatives
• Parent	• Neighbor
• Child	• Friend
• Sibling	• Colleague
• Grandparent	• Parishioner
• Grandchild	• Community volunteer
• Niece/nephew	• Student

The number of caregivers is ever increasing. As more baby boomers enter retirement age, the number of people with limiting illnesses and disabilities also will swell (NFCA, n.d.). Therefore, more people will need to rely on others for assistance. In the past, the typical portrait of a caregiver was a married woman in her forties (NFCA, n.d.). This also will change as life expectancy and divorce rates increase, thus creating a more general picture of who may adopt the role of caregiver.

As the average age of spousal caregivers will increase because of longer life, the age at which children will need to care for their parents will decrease. According to BabyCenter.com (2009), women are waiting longer to start having children, with an average age of 21 in 1970 versus age 25 in 2006. Although this may seem like an increase in age of only a few years over three decades, this just represents the average. More specific data show that more children than ever before are being born to mothers who are age 30 and older (BabyCenter.com, 2009). In addition, 40% of women who seek to adopt are ages 35–39, with the average woman preferring to adopt a child who is two years old or younger (Jones, 2008).

What does this mean for the average caregiver of a parent in the United States? The situation where a child is finishing college (or even high school) just as the parent reaches retirement age will become more common, thereby putting the child in the position of caregiver at a much younger age than ever before. Furthermore, the increasing longevity means that people will be entering retirement and older adulthood and may still have parents who are living well into their 90s or older. The age range, economic status, and position in life will be ever broadening, thereby eliminating a definition for a "typical" caregiver. We can be called upon at any time to fulfill this role.

In addition, the picture of the typical nuclear family is evolving continuously. Children grow up and move out of town. Parents divorce. Same-sex couples with children become more common and accepted in society. Aunts, uncles, and grandparents assume the role of guardian and raise children in a variety of circumstances. Today, "family" comprises not just biologic relationships but also the friends, neighbors, coworkers, former classmates, and fellow church parishioners whom we come to rely on for love and support in the absence of or in addition to a spouse, mother, father, sibling, or other relatives. The bonds with these people sometimes are stronger than any biologic connection. How do they fit in the caregiving profile? What are their rights and responsibilities when a loved one falls ill or has a devastating accident? How do we navigate the sometimes tense family dynamics that were in place before we have the call to duty to serve a loved one in need?

This book is a guide for caregivers as they chaperone a loved one through the challenges of disability and illness. It begins with a primer on in-home care, the usual starting point for caregivers. Next, it will describe options for institutional care as the loved one's need for skilled care increases. Legal and financial issues will be discussed, as well as specific challenges that caregivers may encounter based on their relationship with the person in need. Finally, the appendices feature tips on caregiver and patient safety and many resources for further information and support.

REFERENCES

BabyCenter.com. (2009, August). 22 surprising facts about birth in the United States. Retrieved from http://www.babycenter.com/0_22-surprising-facts-about-birth-in-the-united-states_1372273.bc

Jones, J. (2008). *Adoption experiences of women and men and demand for children to adopt by women 18–44 years of age in the United States, 2002.* Washington, DC: U.S. Department of Health and Human Services.

McLeod, B.W. (Ed.). (2003). *And thou shalt honor: The caregiver's companion.* New York, NY: Rodale.

National Family Caregivers Association. (2000). *Random sample survey of family caregivers.* Unpublished report.

National Family Caregivers Association. (n.d.). Caregiving statistics. Retrieved from http://www.nfcacares.org/who_are_family_caregivers/care_giving_statistics.cfm

U.S. Department of Health and Human Services. (1998). Informal caregiving: Compassion in action. Retrieved from http://aspe.hhs.gov/daltcp/Reports/carebro2.pdf

CHAPTER 2

THE CARE COORDINATOR JOB DESCRIPTION: A HOMECARE PRIMER

INTRODUCTION

If you are reading this book, most likely you are a caregiver already. As mentioned in Chapter 1, a caregiver can be anyone: a 12-year-old who helps his elderly neighbor by shoveling snow, taking out the trash, and mowing the lawn; a retired husband who is dealing with his wife's Alzheimer disease; a young couple with a child who has just been diagnosed with autism; or a sister who moves in with her brother who has been sent home from service in Iraq with head injuries and post-traumatic stress disorder, as well as many others in various stages of life, health, and status.

These people all have one thing in common: they all stepped in to do for their loved ones what their loved ones could not do for themselves. No question that it is a big job, but what exactly are your responsibilities? If your loved one would place an advertisement in the local newspaper for what you do, it would probably look something like this:

Help Wanted: Caregiver

An immediate opening is available for a caregiver. This is an unpaid position.

Responsibilities: Companion, guardian, manager, chauffeur, personal aide, housekeeper, legal aide, social worker, administrative assistant, activities director, accountant, psychologist, spiritual adviser. Must be willing to work long hours with an unpredictable schedule.

Compensation: Bonding between generations, sense of appreciation, increased self-worth, and pride in accomplishments.

Experience not required, and on-the-job training is not provided.

Successful candidates should have good organization skills and a flexible schedule, as well as the ability to provide compassion, security, and comfort to others. Most importantly, the candidate must be able to delegate responsibility to others.

In this chapter, you will learn more about what it means to be a caregiver and, most importantly, whom to ask for help. This chapter will also explore the role of homecare professionals and how to hire one.

A CAREGIVER'S CALL TO SERVICE

As mentioned previously, caregivers do for loved ones what the loved ones cannot do for themselves. Caregivers can be called into service in three basic circumstances:

- Suddenly (accidents, sudden illness such as stroke)

- Instances with limited preparation (learning that a child will be born with Down syndrome)
- Gradually (degenerative diseases such as multiple sclerosis and dementia).

The need for help can fluctuate over time, as in the case of degenerative illnesses, or be temporary, as in the case of caring for a loved one after surgery (U.S. Department of Health and Human Services [DHHS], 2009). In addition, you may be called to serve in a limited capacity (for example, a daughter who is helping with her father's care a few times a week), or you may inherit the role of primary caregiver by undertaking the role full-time. The focus of this book will be those in the primary caregiver position.

Individuals often choose home care for comfort and cost. Some people feel more at ease in their own homes while recuperating from surgery or illness. In addition, receiving care at home costs significantly less than staying at a hospital or rehabilitation center. The costs of homecare services will be discussed in this chapter. For institutional care, see Chapter 3.

THE DUTIES OF A PRIMARY CAREGIVER

In clinical terms, the role of the caregiver is to assist the patient with *activities of daily living*. These are everyday chores that healthy people do without a second thought. People in the early stages of illness and older adults may have difficulty performing household chores, such as cleaning, preparing meals, managing finances and paying bills, tending to their lawn, running errands, driving a car, and doing laundry. As a disease progresses and the patient's mobility or mental capacity decreases, the need for help with self-care will become greater. Self-care duties include moving freely throughout the house (from the bed to a chair in the living room, for example), dressing, using the bathroom, bathing, and feeding oneself.

Examples of Activities of Daily Living

- Personal care: Bathing, dressing, using the toilet, moving about the home, feeding oneself
- Transportation: Driving a car or being able to walk to public transit
- Maintaining a household: Cooking and preparing meals, cleaning, doing laundry, making beds, shopping for groceries and other items, maintaining an automobile
- Clerical tasks: Paying bills, preparing taxes, making doctor's appointments, organizing paperwork and important documents (insurance forms, for example)

A primary family caregiver's job is big essentially because this person is performing the basic activities of two people. Some are taking care of multiple people, thus running several households in addition to their own. They have careers, children, a house of their own to clean and maintain, and community commitments. It is natural to feel overwhelmed, but this is not an unmanageable situation. Sometimes perspective just needs a little adjustment.

First, let's change the job title in the caregiver advertisement to *care coordinator*. From this point forward, you can think of yourself as the person who manages your loved one's care. Managers oversee the tasks that need to be done and step in to perform some of them when needed. Effective care coordinators know how to delegate responsibilities.

In a management position, you will choose the essential duties for which you will be responsible; for example, you may want to handle the legal and financial components of your loved one's care needs. In addition, if your loved one is very modest, he or she may prefer that you help with bathing instead of another person. To begin, make a list with three columns: (a) the activities that your loved one is able to do, (b) the activities that your loved one is able to do with limited supervision, and (c) the activities that your loved one needs help to do. With a highlighter, mark the items in columns b and c that you are willing and able to do. Keep in mind your own physical and time limitations and other responsibilities. For the remaining items, delegate to other relatives, friends, and professional resources. Revisit this list often, as most people will need help for different reasons throughout an illness or recovery period.

Managers do not win a medal for doing it all on their own; in fact, quite the opposite. Care coordinators who insist on doing everything are at risk for burnout, which puts both the coordinator's and the loved one's health at risk. If you take nothing else from this book away with you, make sure you take this: learn to delegate responsibilities.

HOMECARE OPTIONS

As the name suggests, *home care* is when loved ones in need reside within their own residence or the primary caregiver's home, and help with activities of daily living and medical care comes to them. The types of homecare services can be broken down into two categories: unskilled help and skilled help. The goal of home care is to maximize the loved one's independence and functioning (DHHS, 2009).

UNSKILLED HELP

Unskilled service is care that requires little training or education to perform. However, people who perform these duties usually bring a wealth of life experience and compassion. These workers provide help with household chores and perhaps will provide companionship for the loved one while the care coordinator goes to work, tends to other duties, or takes a break (maybe goes to a movie or visits with friends). Unskilled helpers can provide their services for free as volunteers or for a fee. These workers generally are the least expensive people to hire. Although this type of help is considered unskilled, they should be taught some basics about your loved one's needs, such as how to operate equipment in the loved one's home (telephone, television and video equipment, wheelchair, hospital bed), whom to call in an emergency, and where certain items are in the home (drinking glasses, extra blankets, fire extinguisher).

Tasks for Unskilled Help

- Errands: Picking up groceries, dropping off prescriptions and picking up medications, providing transportation to visit relatives, providing transportation to and from doctor's appointments
- Entertainment: Singing, playing a musical instrument, playing games with the patient, sharing a special talent, talking, taking the loved one outdoors for a walk, providing general companionship
- Household chores: Decorating for seasons and special holidays, organizing drawers and closets, dusting, vacuuming, heavy spring cleaning, winterizing the home, preparing meals, loading and unloading a dishwasher, doing laundry, outdoor maintenance such as cleaning gutters, washing windows, and planting flowers
- Personal care: Helping the loved one with hairstyling, manicures, makeup application, and moving about the home

Many creative outlets are available to find unskilled help. Neighbors and friends and their children may be available to provide assistance for free or a nominal fee.

To cast your search net a little wider, many community organizations can be of assistance. Young people have a wealth of energy and compassion that is often overlooked. You can approach youth-oriented groups such as the Boy Scouts, Girl Scouts, and religious youth organizations to consider fulfilling your loved one's needs through a service project. In addition, you can contact the guidance department at a local high school or vocational school. Many high schools require community service hours for graduation and may be able to match you with a student with an interest in the healthcare industry. The students will gain valuable life experience while serving. Local colleges and universities with healthcare and nursing programs also are great sources of help. The people enrolled in these programs already have an interest in providing care, and you will help them to build a résumé of professional experience.

Retired people also are good sources of help and companionship. These individuals often have the time for volunteer work, and it will give them a sense of purpose and fulfillment. If your loved one is an older adult, her friends may be more than willing to help and will already have a common bond with the loved one.

In regard to fee-based services, contact the local Meals-on-Wheels programs to provide hot meals for your loved one (and for yourself, if you qualify). Programs also are available for low-cost transportation to doctor's appointments, physical therapy, shopping, and more. In addition, consult the phone directory for cleaning and lawn care services. In general, professional cleaning and lawn care services will cost more than enlisting the help of a friend or neighbor, but if the job is not performed to your satisfaction, you will have more recourse with an established business than with a volunteer. DHHS (2009) estimates that homemaker services cost an average of $19 per hour. The average cost for a home health aide in the United States is $21 per hour (DHHS, 2009). The total cost of these services would depend on how often the worker visits the home and the type of work performed.

SKILLED HELP

Depending on your loved one's condition, a variety of health professionals, specifically nurses and therapists, are available to make home visits. These professionals provide some of the same services as they would in a hospital setting.

Nurses: Many nursing professionals choose to work in home care. These professionals are from a wide range of educational backgrounds and specialties. When hiring nurses, you need to consider their credentials and level of education. Table 1 describes the basic levels of certification.

Registered nurses can gain credentials in a specialty area that may provide expertise related to your loved one's specific needs. These credentials mean that the nurse has continued his or her education and experience beyond general nursing studies and has knowledge in a particular area. For example, a registered nurse who specializes in cancer nursing may have the OCN® (Oncology Certified Nurse) credential from the Oncology Nursing Certification Corporation. The nurse's résumé or curriculum vitae will list details about credentials.

The cost of home nursing care varies with the experience and education of the nurse, whether the nurse is an independent care provider or is hired from an agency, and the level of care provided.

Table 1. Nursing Professionals by Job Title			
Job Title	**Education/ Training**	**Certification**	**Basic Duties**
Home health aides/ personal homecare aides	On-the-job training Requirements vary by state.	Must participate in basic program and complete certification for Medicare/Medicaid reimbursement	Perform basic housekeeping, home sanitation, safety, and emergency response Help patient to eat, dress, and bathe
Nursing aides/ psychiatric aides	High school diploma	Certified Nurse's Assistant (CNA) Requirements vary by state.	Help patient to eat, dress, and bathe Take vital signs (blood pressure, pulse, respirations) and report changes to nursing/ medical staff Psychiatric aides help with personal hygiene, socialization, and recreation.
Licensed practical nurses (LPNs) (also known as licensed vocational nurses)	One year of training at state-approved vocational/ technical school or community college	National Council Licensure Examination for Practical Nurses (NCLEX-PN)	Same duties as a nursing aide, plus provide basic bedside care, prepare and give injections and enemas, dress wounds, monitor catheters, collect samples for laboratory testing, and administer medication under the supervision of a registered nurse

(Continued on next page)

	Education/		
Table 1. Nursing Professionals by Job Title (Continued)			
Job Title	**Training**	**Certification**	**Basic Duties**
Registered nurses	Diploma from an approved school of nursing (three years) Associate's degree (two to three years) Bachelor's degree (four years) Master's degree	National Council Licensure Examination for Registered Nurses (NCLEX-RN) Optional advanced practice certification based on specialty Additional credentials and certification per specialty based on portfolio of experience and/or continuing education credits	Administer medication, hang IVs, insert and remove catheters, assist physicians, and develop and manage care plans. More specific duties based on specialty. Often oversee LPNs and aides.

Note. Based on information from U.S. Bureau of Labor Statistics, 2009.

An important consideration when looking for skilled nursing care is what the nurse is allowed to do based on her credentials and certification. For example, in some states, licensed practical nurses (referred to as LPNs) are not allowed to hang IV bags or administer medications without supervision by a registered nurse (U.S. Bureau of Labor Statistics, 2009). Your loved one's physician or social worker can help you to determine the level of care needed, as well as the type of skilled nursing professional that is appropriate for your situation.

Therapists: A variety of rehabilitation therapists will be available to your loved one, depending on the condition and situation. Here are some examples:

- Occupational therapists help clients improve their independence by teaching them to adapt to their home and work environment in the context of their illness or disability.
- Physical therapists work with clients to achieve the highest level of mobility and function after an injury or illness. For individuals who are born with disabilities, physical therapists help them reach their full potential for movement and functionality.
- Respiratory therapists provide care that helps people with lung disease and difficulty breathing.
- Speech therapists help clients with oral communication difficulties, such as a child with a developmental delay or a person who is recovering from a stroke or traumatic brain injury.
- Mental health therapists teach clients coping mechanisms for problems caused by illness or injury. In addition, these professionals work with emotional and cognitive issues associated with developmental and congenital (the part of the brain that deals with awareness, memory, reasoning, and judgment) illnesses.

These services are available in the home, at an outpatient facility by appointment, or a combination of the two. Most likely, the physician or social worker will request these services for your loved one, so you will not need to search on your own. However, if you desire extra help, ask the social worker or physician what resources are available. Health insurance or Medicaid covers many of these services. See Chapter 4 for an overview of payment options for in-home services such as therapy and skilled nursing care.

SOCIAL WORKERS' ROLE IN HOME CARE

Social workers are another type of skilled personnel who will help you to coordinate your loved one's care. Social workers will act as an advocate on your loved one's behalf to find the services needed for care (National Association of Social Workers [NASW], n.d.). The social worker may meet with you and your loved one at the bedside in the hospital or may visit you at your home. Services of a social worker are usually provided through a hospital, nonprofit organization, or state or federal agency.

Social workers are professionals who coordinate the many components of healthcare and social services. These professionals will help you contact agencies, can arrange for housing or transportation if needed, and will help you create a plan of care for your loved one and assemble all the necessary components to achieve that care. Social workers will follow up with you to monitor your progress and adjust the care plan if necessary. Most importantly, they educate and empower patients and caregivers (NASW, n.d.). Other names for social workers are case manager and information and referral specialist.

HOW TO HIRE HEALTHCARE PERSONNEL

Now that you know the variety of skilled help available, the next step is to assess exactly what type of services you need. If your loved one will have the disability for the remainder of life, you will need to reassess the need on a regular basis according to your loved one's health status. A social worker can help you determine what kind of skilled help you need.

The two most common ways to hire a skilled nursing professional is either independently or through an agency (MetLife & National Alliance for Caregiving, 2007). You will have to weigh factors of need, finances, and personal preferences to choose the best route. Table 2 provides some general considerations. Regardless of where the skilled nursing professional is from, you and your loved one should meet with the professional to talk about his or her skills and your expectations. Although using an agency to hire healthcare personnel requires less research on each individual candidate, you should always research the reputability of the agency by contacting your local Better Business Bureau, asking others for recommendations, and consulting with your loved one's physician or social worker.

Table 2. Hiring Skilled Help From an Agency Versus Hiring an Individual		
Concern	**Agency Hire**	**Individual Hire**
Cost	Generally higher than private hiring	Generally lower than hiring through an agency
Convenience	Agency prescreens applicants and provides clearances and background checks. Caregiver and patient only need to be concerned about personality. Agency pays the health professional and is responsible for taxes and other employment issues.	Caregiver can choose from friends and family members whom both the patient and caregiver know. Caregiver is responsible for conducting criminal background checks, interviewing potential candidates, and checking references. Caregivers as employers of workers or independent contractors may have responsibilities regarding taxes.
		(Continued on next page)

Table 2. Hiring Skilled Help From an Agency Versus Hiring an Individual *(Continued)*		
Concern	**Agency Hire**	**Individual Hire**
Reliability	A system is in place to send a replacement in case of call-offs.	Caregiver would be responsible for finding a replacement if the individual does not report to work.
Job function	Ideal for hiring skilled nursing professionals	Ideal for hiring unskilled personnel, such as personal assistants, nighttime companions, and people to perform housekeeping and maintenance duties.

Some important questions to ask an agency:

- Is your agency insured and bonded? (*Bonded* means that the agency has a type of policy that will pay the client in the event that the agency is unable to perform the agreed-upon duties.)
- What are your rates?
- Are any of the services covered by my loved one's health insurance?
- Will you help with processing Medicare, Medicaid, and health insurance claims?
- What is your policy for when a nurse calls off? How quickly will replacement staff be available?
- What is your average employee turnover?
- What is the interview process? Will we be able to select a nurse, or will we be assigned whoever is available?
- What happens if my loved one has a personality conflict with the nurse? Will we have the option to switch to someone else?
- Will my loved one have a primary care provider, or will the personnel rotate? How often will the nurses rotate, such as every day or on weekends?

Important questions to ask a nurse include the following:
- How long have you been a nurse?
- Where else have you worked? What kind of experience do you have?
- Do you have experience with my loved one's condition?
- What kind of certification do you have?
- What is your availability?
- Do you smoke?
- Why did you become a nurse?

Of course, you will need to follow up with details on a résumé, such as contacting previous employers and schools, and conduct your own background check if you are hiring an independent caregiver. Contact your local police department for instruction on how to do this. Also, many private investigation companies offer background check services to employers.

It is very important to note that as an employer, you may be responsible for Social Security and other taxes. In addition, if you hire a person as an independent contractor, you may be responsible for reporting the amount of money paid within a year to that individual, and he will be required to claim that payment as earned income. If you pay an individual more than $600 in a tax year, you will be required to provide that person with a 1099 form (Internal Revenue Service, 2010). To do this, you will need to have the individual complete a W-9 form to obtain his taxpayer identification number (Internal Revenue Service, 2007). Consult with a professional tax preparer or accountant for tax-related details. This applies not only to independent nurse caregivers but also to other employees that you may pay directly, such as a housekeeper or gardener. (This is not the case if you are paying for the services of an agency or business that acts as the employer for the workers.) In regard to informal caregivers, it is best to contact an accountant in your state to clarify your responsibilities in reporting payments made to neighbors, friends, family, and others who are paid for their services.

RESPITE CARE

Respite is a short break. Respite care is available so that both the caregiver and the loved one can have some time apart from one another to rest and to interact with other people. The break can be as little as a few hours, overnight, for a weekend, or for a week or two. The cost of professional respite care can range from $15–$25 per hour (Elderlycareservices.org, 2009). This care can be received in the home or at centers outside the home.

ADULT DAY CARE

Adult day care is a service provided by many public, private, nonprofit, and for-profit organizations. Centers usually are open Monday through Friday during typical business hours (Rose, Segal, & White, 2007). In addition to allowing the caregiver to work and relax, adult daycare centers provide socialization and a reason to leave the home every day. Other benefits include mental and physical stimulation.

Depending on the center, some activities include arts and crafts, games, musical entertainment, light exercise, and local outings. Adults who can benefit from this service include people with intellectual disabilities, older adults who have some physical limitations, and individuals in the early stages of Alzheimer disease or dementia (Rose et al., 2007).

CAMP OUTINGS

Another form of respite care involves disease- or disability-specific outings for adults and children and their family caregivers. Most of these are run by nonprofit organizations and foundations and are offered either for free or at a minimal cost. A social worker can help you connect with organizations that provide these services. You also can search for local and regional groups on the Internet and contact them directly for information about their services.

Respite camp events can take the form of a day camp or sleep-away camp. Some involve the whole family, whereas others are just for the person with the disability or illness. Activities usually focus on typical summer camp experiences, including horseback riding, campfires, crafts, swimming, and boating. Of course, each activity is adapted for full participation by all campers.

Camps for families can provide a getaway from a hectic world and promote bonding between family members with activities that involve the whole family. Separate activities offer personal growth and development for children with disabilities and their siblings (United Cerebral Palsy, n.d.). Some camps offer parents a chance to relax with golf, massages, and outdoor activities, with their children being close and well supervised (United Cerebral Palsy, n.d.). Caregivers and siblings also can meet with their peers for education and support (Wayne & White, 2010).

A WORD ABOUT SAFETY

Another beginning step as you coordinate the care for your loved one is to assess your living situation. Now is a good time to take a safety inventory of the home where your loved one will be living.

- Ensure that the electrical service is up to code and well maintained, especially if your loved one will be using medical equipment that depends on electricity. Ask an electrician if the service can handle the extra energy draw.

- Make an appointment with a heating and cooling technician to inspect the furnace. Spring, summer, and early fall are good times to do this because furnace specialists are the least busy and sometimes offer special inspection and cleaning packages.
- If the furnace does break in the winter, move your loved one to another location until it is repaired. Do not rely on an oven, portable heater, or fireplace for heat, especially if your loved one uses oxygen therapy. These alternative heat sources are fire hazards and increase the risk of carbon monoxide poisoning. Households that include an individual who is on oxygen therapy need to be especially cautious because oxygen is highly flammable, and the pressurized tanks are an explosion hazard.
- To avoid a significant fire hazard, quit smoking, and do not allow your loved one to smoke. Under no circumstances should your loved one be allowed to smoke while in bed or on soft furniture such as a sofa or recliner. This is particularly important for people on oxygen therapy.
- Install smoke and carbon monoxide detectors and place all-purpose fire extinguishers in strategic areas in the home. If your loved one is deaf, hearing impaired, or perhaps a sound sleeper because of illness or medication, systems are available that use vibration or strobe lights in addition to an audible siren.
- Rid the home of trip and fall hazards such as loose electrical cords, throw rugs, and excessive furniture. Install handrails where practical, especially in stairways and bathrooms. Use antislip mats and shower chairs in the bathtub.
- Move commonly used items to lower shelves.

More safety suggestions are available in Appendix 1.

POINTS TO REMEMBER

- Delegating responsibilities will make your job as care coordinator much easier.
- Look to people in the community to provide help with activities of daily living.
- Young people are often an untapped resource.
- Be aware of the types of skilled nursing professionals available, as well as their abilities and limitations based on their education and certification.
- You can either hire an independent nursing professional or use an agency.
- Adult day care and formal respite care are available to lessen the burden.
- Assess the home for potential safety hazards.

REFERENCES

Elderlycareservices.org. (2009, October 7). The cost of respite care [Blog]. Retrieved from http://www.elderlycareservices.org/wordpress/index.php/2009/10/07/the-cost-of-respite-care

Internal Revenue Service. (2007, October). Request for taxpayer number and certification. Retrieved from http://www.irs.gov/pub/irs-pdf/fw9.pdf

Internal Revenue Service. (2010). Instructions for Form 1099-MISC. Retrieved from http://www.irs.gov/pub/irs-pdf/i1099msc.pdf

MetLife & National Alliance for Caregiving. (2007). SinceYouCare®: Family caregiving. Retrieved from http://www.metlife.com/assets/cao/mmi/publications/since-you-care-guides/mmi-family-caregiving.pdf

National Association of Social Workers. (n.d.). About social workers. Retrieved from http://www.helpstartshere.org/about-social-workers

Rose, A., Segal, J., & White, M. (2007, March). Adult day care centers: Finding the best center for your needs. Retrieved from http://www.helpguide.org/elder/adult_day_care_centers.htm#authors

United Cerebral Palsy. (n.d.). What is respite care? Retrieved from http://www.ucp.org/ucp_channeldoc.cfm/1/11/51/51-51/2106

U.S. Bureau of Labor Statistics. (2009). Occupational outlook handbook (2010–2011 ed.). Retrieved from http://www.bls.gov/OCO

U.S. Department of Health and Human Services. (2009, December). National clearinghouse for long-term care information. Retrieved from http://www.longtermcare.gov/LTC/Main_site/Paying_LTC/Costs_Of_Care/Costs_Of_Care.aspx

Wayne, M., & White, M. (2009, January 9). Respite care: Finding and choosing services and providers. Retrieved from http://www.helpguide.org/elder/respite_care.htm#authors

CHAPTER 3

INSTITUTIONAL CARE OPTIONS

INTRODUCTION

For this chapter, we are going back to basics. Everyone at some point in their lives has either been to the hospital to receive care or to visit someone there. But, if you are not in the healthcare industry, have you ever thought about what the purpose of a hospital is? You may drive past a rehabilitation center on your way to work every day, but have you thought about what goes on in there?

Words like *nursing home, hospice,* and *group home* are scary for both patients and their families. Older loved ones may have memories of dimly lit, crowded hospitals and care facilities where their grandparents or other loved ones may have spent their remaining days. Mental hospitals and facilities for people with intellectual and emotional disabilities may conjure up images out of *One Flew Over the Cuckoo's Nest* or *Shutter Island* of cold nurses and electric shock treatments.

A clear understanding of the services that these institutions provide will help both you and your loved one feel more at ease about using them. Technology and philosophies about patient care have come a long way from the stark, windowless healthcare and mental health facilities of the early 20th century. Also, attitudes about placing a loved one in one of these institutions are a matter of perspective, which will be discussed in this chapter.

HOSPITALS

Hospitals are such an integral part of society that many people probably do not stop and think about the philosophy behind them. Of course, most people know that the hospital is for medical treatment, surgeries, and emergency care. At one time, the community hospital was one building that provided diagnostics, emergency care, critical care, surgery, labor and delivery services, rehabilitation, and hospice care. However, as medical technology and the healthcare industry evolved, the hospital as a single entity has transitioned to a complex campus-style health system. These institutions and their purpose are often misunderstood. Some people may fear them as "germ factories." Others may feel they were "kicked out" when they were transferred from the hospital to a nursing home or rehabilitation center or sent home to receive further care or rehabilitation therapy. This section will explain some of the services that hospitals offer and will define levels of care, including acute, intensive, outpatient, and chronic. In addition, this chapter will suggest ways to find a hospital that provides the best care in your loved one's area.

BASIC SERVICES

The general menu of hospital offerings includes emergency care, surgery, diagnostics (for example, blood tests, x-rays, urine tests), and short-term hospitalization (McKenzie, n.d.). Some hospitals specialize in one particular area, such as mental health, pediatrics, or women's health, whereas some larger hospitals will have units or floors devoted to these and other specialized services. As mentioned previously, a hospital can be part of a much larger integrated system of medical practices, rehabilitation facilities, and outpatient care centers. Therefore, the same health system could include a large central campus of buildings with many satellite offices and facilities distributed over a wide region.

Acute care refers to short-term medical care for serious disease (such as heart attack, stroke, or severe breathing problems) or trauma (such as broken bones or head injuries) (Merriam-Webster, n.d.). This type of care also refers to care immediately after surgery and emergency services (sometimes called *urgent care*).

Intensive care (also called *critical care*) is a form of acute care that involves highly focused treatment and observation that takes place in a separate unit of the hospital (U.S. National Library of Medicine & National Institutes of Health, 2009). This area usually has a lower staff-to-patient ratio, meaning the number of patients assigned to one healthcare professional is much lower, perhaps two or three patients to one nurse compared to five or six patients to one nurse in other areas in the hospital.

AMBULATORY CARE

The average length of stay in a hospital has steadily decreased from an average of 7.3 days in 1980 to 4.6 days in 2007 (Agency for Healthcare Research and Quality, 2007; Centers for Disease Control and Prevention [CDC], 2001). This trend can be attributed to the growing number of outpatient, or *ambulatory care*, services that hospitals provide. Procedures and therapies that used to require hospitalization, such as rehabilitation therapy, dialysis treatment, chemotherapy, IV antibiotics, and urinary catheterization, can be safely and efficiently performed on an outpatient basis and monitored by home-care nurses (CDC, 2001). In addition, medical technology has resulted in more efficient and less-invasive surgical techniques that shorten recovery time.

FINDING THE BEST HOSPITAL CARE

You and your loved one can be proactive about where to go for treatment. Of course, in an emergency, the ambulance personnel will take your loved one to the closest location, but otherwise, choices are available. Many doctors are affiliated with several hospitals and healthcare systems, and health insurance policies often provide flexibility as to where a person can receive care. Not all hospitals are created equal or designed to give the best treatment for your loved one's condition.

Guidelines for Choosing a Hospital

- Does my loved one's health insurance cover care at this hospital?
- Does my loved one's physician have permission to admit patients at this hospital? If not, is my loved one willing to change doctors?
- What is the hospital's record of experience with my loved one's condition? (Ask the hospital about statistics regarding the number of patients with the same or similar condition admitted to the hospital or who are undergoing a similar procedure and patient outcomes.)
- How does the hospital monitor care quality?
- What is the hospital's status with the Joint Commission (an independent nonprofit organization that provides healthcare organizations with certification and accreditation)? You can find information about specific hospitals by visiting www.qualitycheck.org/consumer/searchQCR.aspx, or you can get a free report by calling 1-630-792-5800.

Note. Based on information from Agency for Healthcare Research and Quality, n.d.; Joint Commission, n.d.

REHABILITATION CENTERS

Rehabilitation centers are usually stand-alone facilities that offer both outpatient and inpatient therapies after illness or injury. Other types of rehabilitation centers focus on addiction recovery and emotional and mental health disorders. The main focus of these facilities is to help patients regain their independence. They may offer physical, occupational, and speech therapies, as well as counseling to help with problem solving, adjusting to new physical challenges, and coping with a chronic condition or a slow recovery process. Inpatient stays are usually limited to when the patient reaches certain recovery goals. Some patients, especially those of advanced age, will transition to a nursing home at this stage.

LONG-TERM CARE FACILITIES

Long-term care facilities offer patients personal and medical assistance based on age, level of mobility, and severity of illness or disability. Although separate terms exist to describe the level of care (such as *nursing home, assisted living, independent living,* or *hospice*), some institutions are structured so that the patient will be able to transition to a higher level of care without much disruption. The patient may be able to remain in the same room or just move to a different area of the facility when more skilled care and observation is required. This section describes the different types of facilities to consider when a loved one may need or desire long-term care outside the home. Your loved one's social worker or physician can help you assess the level of care and attention that your loved one will need. Here are some things to look for when visiting and shopping for a facility after you determine what type of facility is best for your loved one.

Guidelines for Touring a Residential Care Facility

A tour of a residential care facility can be an overwhelming experience. As you tour a residential facility, make notes about what you see, hear, and smell. Later, you can compare your notes on each facility.

Location
- How close is the facility to the nearest hospital? Fire department?
- How far is it from your home?
- What is the neighborhood like?

The Building
- Are the road, driveway, and parking lot well maintained?
- Does the facility have adequate parking?
- Is the landscaping well maintained (the grass is cut, no leaves or other debris is on the sidewalks)?
- Does the building seem to be in general good repair?
- When you walk inside, does it smell clean?
- As you walk through each area of the facility, are they neat and uncluttered?
- Do the floors and other surfaces seem clean?
- Are the bathrooms clean and stocked with paper products?
- Are the trash cans emptied? If applicable, are there separate containers for biohazard waste?
- Do you see first aid kits, fire extinguishers, and automatic external defibrillators?
- Are fire exits well marked and unblocked by furniture or equipment?
- Does it seem crowded with people? Do the residents seem to have enough space for personal belongings and medical equipment?

(Continued on next page)

Guidelines for Touring a Residential Care Facility
(Continued)

The Personnel
- Are nurses and other support staff visible? What is the patient-to-caregiver ratio?
- Do the people who work there seem attentive? Are they interacting with the residents?
- In general, do the employees seem happy?

The Residents
- Do the residents seem content?
- Is the residents' personal hygiene generally good (such as clean clothes, combed hair, clean faces and hands)?
- Are the residents interacting with each other? Do they seem busy and engaged in activities?

Activities
- What type of group activities does the facility offer, such as games, parties, and arts and crafts?
- How often do outside community services visit, such as a library book cart or local religious groups?
- Does the facility have therapy animals? This will be especially comforting to loved ones who had to leave a pet behind or who have fond memories of pets or growing up on a farm. Many facilities will have cats wandering about to comfort the residents, and others will have local humane agencies visit with dogs (sometimes even miniature horses or potbellied pigs).
- Does the facility provide outings for shopping or entertainment?

INDEPENDENT LIVING AND CONGREGATE CARE

Independent living housing is an option for older adults who are able to perform most activities of daily living. This type of residence provides a community environment, usually with a common area for parties and social activities. Some amenities include laundry and housekeeping services and security personnel. Most independent living facilities require the residents to prepare their own meals and to shop for themselves. Some residents are still able to drive, whereas others will rely on relatives, a provided shuttle service, or public transportation to grocery shop, attend church, or go to doctor's appointments.

Congregate care is very similar to independent living. The difference is that congregate care features more communal living. These facilities include a common dining area.

GROUP HOMES

A group home is a small residential facility that serves children or adults who require special care that limits their ability to live alone. Group homes can provide care for people with intellectual or developmental disabilities, individuals with physical disabilities, people recovering from substance and alcohol abuse, children who are victims of abuse and neglect, or people who are homeless and are reintegrating into society. These facilities usually have six or fewer residents with similar needs and are staffed 24 hours a day by trained caregivers (Friedrich, n.d.).

A group home situation is a good opportunity for young adults with social, emotional, or intellectual disabilities to gain some independence from their parents in a supervised environment. Caregivers and counselors teach life skills, such as personal hygiene and maintaining a household, as well as how to build relationships, solve problems, and resolve conflicts. Residents have responsibilities matched to the level of their physical and intellectual capabilities, which fosters a sense of community and purpose.

Some group homes are temporary placements where residents can then transition into an independent living situation or return to their family. Other placements are long term or permanent (Friedrich, n.d.).

ASSISTED LIVING

Assisted living centers offer apartment-style living with the option for a higher level of care than if the individual were living independently. This option is for people who need less skilled nursing care than people who are in a nursing home but may need help with meals and medication (this involves an additional charge). This type of facility acts as a bridge between independent living and a nursing home. The national average for the monthly cost of care in an assisted living facility is $3,131 (U.S. Department of Health and Human Services [DHHS], 2009). This does not include services such as housekeeping, laundry, and other amenities, which are often offered for an additional fee.

NURSING HOMES

Nursing homes are residential facilities that provide skilled nursing care and focus on improving quality of life and personal independence. Residents usually are older adults, but some younger residents also may live in a nursing home if they require special care because of intellectual disabilities, mental illness, or physical and developmental disabilities. Some residents also may be at these facilities temporarily if home care for a serious illness or injury is not an option. These facilities can be associated with a hospital, health system, or retirement community, or they can be independently owned and operated.

In addition to skilled nursing, nursing homes provide the following amenities:

- Pharmacy services
- On-staff physicians or physicians from an affiliated hospital who make regular "rounds"
- Wheelchairs, scooters, and patient lifts
- Specialized medical equipment

- Access to physical and other types of therapies
- Access to mental health and spiritual counseling
- Meal plans tailored to the client's preferences and nutritional needs, such as low-salt, diabetic, kosher, or vegetarian diets.

Depending on the facility, some specialized services, such as dialysis, can be performed on site, or the facility will arrange for transportation to hospitals or specialized treatment clinics.

In 2009, the average cost of a semiprivate room in a nursing home was $198 per day, and a private room was $219 per day (DHHS, 2009). Depending on the facility, the cost can be subsidized entirely or in part by Medicare, Medicaid, or long-term care insurance. See Chapter 5 for more about paying for long-term care.

HOSPICE AND PALLIATIVE CARE

Although separate facilities exist for end-of-life care, *hospice* is more of a care philosophy rather than a tangible building. Hospice care can occur in a center specially designated to this service, a special section of a nursing home, at the hospital, or even in the home. This type of care is for patients with limited life expectancy when all curative treatment possibilities have been exhausted. Patients are usually in hospice care for six months or less (Center to Advance Palliative Care, n.d.).

The focus of hospice care is quality of life. This means that the patient is kept as comfortable as possible, and invasive treatments and procedures are not performed. However, this does not mean that the patient will lack professional attention. A multidisciplinary team, including physicians, nurses, a social worker, a counselor, and a spiritual adviser work together to help the patient and family through the end-of-life transition (Homant, 2002).

Palliative (pa-lee-uh-tiv) care is "the medical specialty focused on relief of the pain, stress, and other debilitation symptoms of serious illness" (Center to Advance Palliative Care, n.d., para. 1). This type of care is provided in the hospice setting but also can start much earlier in the healthcare process. Palliative care can be offered in conjunction with aggressive treatments that aim to cure the patient. Palliative approaches usually are used to treat symptoms that are caused by the natural progression of an illness or treatment for that illness, such as shortness of breath, fatigue, constipation, lack of appetite, and pain. It is important to note that the purpose of palliative and end-of-life care *is not* to speed up the process of dying, nor is it to prolong suffering in order to extend life (Pace & Mann, 2008).

LETTING GO

Sometimes, the loved one's condition, age, or health status is to the point where it is beyond the care coordinator's available skills, abilities, and time. In addition, the care coordinator's own health and physical and emotional abilities may decline. Some care coordinators may feel like they are disappointing their loved one or that they are "sending their loved one away" when the time comes that a residential facility is the best option. It is important to consider all family relationships, job demands, personal health, and goals. The job of care coordinator is a demanding one, but these demands should not come before your well-being. Many emotions can be attached to the decision to move a loved one into a residential care facility. Some loved ones may resist going to the hospital because they fear that they may never come home again, or they may have negative memories of visiting people in nursing homes many years ago.

Care coordinators should take comfort in the decision to choose a residential facility because these places are designed to provide patients with security and skilled care that allow for maximum independence and quality of life. In addition, residential facilities provide them with socialization with a group of peers who have had similar experiences and face similar challenges.

For example, if a care coordinator is a parent of a child with intellectual disabilities who has reached adulthood, the parent may feel as if he is giving up on the child by placing him to live in a group home. However, a shift in perspective would actually allow the parent to see that the child would have a similar degree of independence as siblings and friends who have gone away to college. The child will be able to live with other young adults, create bonds and friendships outside the family, and perhaps train for a job that would provide pride and fulfillment. He could learn important life skills and responsibilities by helping to maintain the household by doing chores and helping the resident adviser with grocery shopping and meal preparation.

Adult children who are in the position of placing their parents in a nursing home also may feel guilty about the decision. However, they can be reassured that their parents will receive around-the-clock care that the children are unable to give. As care coordinators weigh the options for loved ones, researching the local facilities and services will provide peace of mind for both the care coordinator and the loved one. This knowledge will not only help to find the best care options available but also will give the whole family confidence that the best decision has been made for the loved one's well-being.

POINTS TO REMEMBER

- The healthcare industry's philosophy of care has evolved from independent hospitals and physician's practices into very complex integrated health systems.
- The average hospital stay is much shorter than it was in 1980. This is not only because of cost-saving measures but also because of more efficient technologies and less-invasive procedures that speed up recovery time.
- Many options are available for residential care outside the home. A good fit for your loved one can be made based on your loved one's specific needs, including level of independence, severity of disability or illness, and personal preferences.
- Many emotions can be tied to choosing a residential facility, but doing research and visiting facilities together and discussing your loved one's goals, abilities, and ideas about quality of life can help ease the transition and reassure everyone that the loved one will receive the best care.

REFERENCES

Agency for Healthcare Research and Quality. (2007). HCUPnet: National and regional estimates on hospital use for all patients from the HCUP nationwide inpatient sample (NIS). Retrieved from http://hcupnet.ahrq.gov/HCUPnet.jsp

Agency for Healthcare Research and Quality. (n.d.). Choosing a hospital. Retrieved from http://www.ahrq.gov/consumer/qnt/qnthosp.htm

Center to Advance Palliative Care. (n.d.). What is palliative care? Retrieved from http://www.getpalliativecare.org/whatis

Centers for Disease Control and Prevention. (2001, April 24). Hospital stays grow shorter, heart disease leading cause of hospitalization [Press release]. Retrieved from http://www.cdc.gov/media/pressrel/r010427b.htm

Friedrich, S.L. (n.d.). Group homes. *Encyclopedia of mental disorders.* Retrieved from http://www.minddisorders.com/Flu-Inv/Group-homes.html

Homant, S.F. (2002). Hospice care. In K.K. Kuebler & P. Esper (Eds.), *Palliative practices from A–Z for the bedside clinician* (pp. 147–150). Pittsburgh, PA: Oncology Nursing Society.

Joint Commission. (n.d.). About the Joint Commission. Retrieved from http://www.jointcommission.org/AboutUs

McKenzie, N. (n.d.). Hospital services. *Encyclopedia of surgery.* Retrieved from http://www.surgeryencyclopedia.com/Fi-La/Hospital-Services.html

Merriam-Webster. (n.d.). Acute care. Retrieved from http://www.merriam-webster.com/medical/acute%20care

Pace, J.C., & Mann, C. (2008). Palliative care. In P. Esper & K.K. Kuebler (Eds.), *Palliative practices from A–Z for the bedside clinician* (2nd ed., pp. 211–215). Pittsburgh, PA: Oncology Nursing Society.

U.S. Department of Health and Human Services. (2009, December). National clearinghouse for long-term care information. Retrieved from http://www.longtermcare.gov/LTC/Main_site/Paying_LTC/Costs_Of_Care/Costs_Of_Care.aspx

U.S. National Library of Medicine & National Institutes of Health. (2009). Critical care. Retrieved from http://www.nlm.nih.gov/medlineplus/criticalcare.html

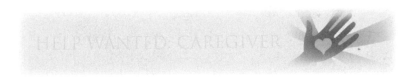

CHAPTER 4

HELP WANTED: LEGAL AIDE

INTRODUCTION

When assuming responsibility for your loved one's decisions, many legal terms will begin to pop up, such as *proxy, advance directive,* and *power of attorney.* This chapter will introduce you to some of them. It is important to note that laws vary by state. For a complete understanding of your loved one's rights, your responsibilities, and other legal issues, it is best to seek the advice of a professional such as an attorney or legal adviser. A social worker can put you in touch with these services.

BECOMING THE DECISION MAKER

Many legal terms describe someone who makes the decisions for another person when that person cannot, including *representative, agent, proxy,* and *attorney-in-fact.* They all mean basically the same thing: the law acknowledges that this person has the right to make decisions on another's behalf. As a patient's representative, the proxy will have the rights to receive medical information, review the medical record, ask questions, request second opinions, and consult with the medical team about treatment options (American Bar Association [ABA] Commission on Law and Aging, n.d.). The medical team will look to the proxy to authorize transfers to another institution or another physician and provide consent or refusal for treatment or tests (ABA Commission on Law and Aging, n.d.).

ADVANCE DIRECTIVES

A person can become a proxy in two ways: either by court appointment or by the patient's choice. The patient can make his wishes legally binding by filing an advance directive. An advance directive is a legal document that states a person's wishes regarding medical treatment in the event that the person is unable to make these decisions on his own. The document will usually include a section that appoints a proxy and an alternative proxy in case the first is unwilling or unable to fulfill the duties of the role. This document also may describe the patient's ideals regarding quality of life, pain control, and life-sustaining treatments. Covered items could include being placed on a respirator, receiving nutrition or hydration, and treating illnesses with medication when swallowing becomes impossible, as well as the person's wishes regarding autopsy and organ donation in the event of death.

Ideally, the person who is appointed proxy will know well ahead of time and can have a detailed discussion with the patient about her wishes, ideas about what it means to have a "good death," and what the proxy should do in specific scenarios related to the patient's illness. The proxy should read the advance directive carefully and ask questions if any items are unclear. If the patient is unable to communicate at this point, the proxy should consult both the patient's lawyer and physician for clarification.

Sometimes, being a proxy puts you in a difficult position. You may not agree with your loved one's wishes or choices, and following them may seem to make his condition worse. It is important to respect the wishes of your loved one but also to actively seek support of the team around you; social workers, physicians, clergy, nurses, and psychologists have the experience to offer you professional advice and to ease your fears and concerns. The proxy's job is to support the loved one's requests while keeping him comfortable. The best way to do this is to actively consult with the healthcare team to make informed decisions based on your loved one's wishes.

LIVING WILL

A living will can be either part of an advance directive or a separate document. This document outlines the patient's wishes for medical treatment, especially life-sustaining therapies related to breathing, food, and hydration. It is invoked only when the patient is in a permanent unconscious state, has permanent severe brain damage, or is terminally ill (Caritas Good Samaritan Medical Center, n.d.).

If possible, consult with your loved one and the physician to review this document as soon as possible. What does "no intervention" or "no invasive treatment" mean to them? Terminology may mean something different to your loved one than it does in standard medical practice. The physician can explain what treatments are available, what to expect throughout the course of disease, and what typically happens at the end of life. These are important things to consider before your loved one is unable to communicate.

DO-NOT-RESUSCITATE ORDER

A do-not-resuscitate (DNR) order is similar to a living will in that it allows the patient to specify limitations on the types of treatment that the patient receives. It is a signed form that is kept in the patient's medical record and will be invoked if the patient goes into cardiac arrest (the patient stops breathing and his or her heart stops beating). This document states that if this situation occurs, the patient does not want the doctor or rescue personnel to take any measures to restart breathing or get the heart to start beating again, such as defibrillation or cardiopulmonary resuscitation (CPR). This type of document is usually signed when the patient is in the final stages of illness when CPR will only temporarily delay death.

If the patient is in the hospital and *DNR* is clearly marked on the patient's chart, this is usually not an area of controversy. However, if the patient is at home, home healthcare workers need to be made aware of the situation. In addition, if paramedics are called, they also must be informed that the patient has signed a DNR order because paramedics are legally required to provide rescue treatment, including CPR, unless presented with the signed order. The proxy can help make the wishes of the patient known by providing copies of the DNR order to the home healthcare agency, notifying all healthcare personnel of the decision, and placing a copy of the DNR order and a sign by the loved one's bed so that it will be easy to access in the event that emergency personnel arrive at the home.

OTHER IMPORTANT LEGAL DOCUMENTS

Other important legal documents include a will, living trust (sometimes called a revocable trust), and a durable power of attorney for finances. Most people are familiar with a will as a document instructing how a person's possessions are to be dispersed after the person's death and who will become the guardian of any minor children. A living trust is similar to a will in that it states a person's wishes about how property and finances should be handled (Iowa State Bar Association, 2004). This document allows for transfer of property and money to a trustee, who will use it to maintain a person's estate and to care for any minor children in the event that the person is unable to manage his own finances.

A durable power of attorney for finances is similar to a durable power of attorney for health care. It is a document that appoints a financial decision maker in the event that a person is incapacitated. All of these documents have similarities and subtle differences. Each state has its own rules for how these documents are set up. It is important for your loved one to consult a lawyer who specializes in estate planning in order to properly document these decisions.

These documents are important to you as the care coordinator because if you are named as trustee or durable power of attorney for finances, you will have control over your loved one's financial resources. This will allow you to pay for the patient's medical and other expenses before choosing to dip into your own savings. Without this control, access to certain accounts, such as pensions and savings, could be delayed or denied, placing both you and your loved one in financial jeopardy.

Assuming financial responsibility for another person's accounts should be done carefully in order to protect your own financial condition. Situations vary, but in general, you are to act as manager, not co-signer or guarantor (someone who promises to pay a debt when another cannot), and your accounts and all transactions should remain separate so that it remains a choice—not a legal obligation—to use your own funds when your loved one's estate is depleted (Repa, n.d.; Steinberg, n.d.).

However, if you are living in a home or are using property, such as a car, that is only in your loved one's name, you must investigate if that property can be seized to settle debts or to pay nursing home fees, and if transferring the property title or deed to your name will prevent this from happening. In this case, it is especially vital that everything is in order within the proper time frame, or you risk losing the property.

In addition, other documents such as a birth certificate, Social Security card, and military papers are important for both family and unrelated care coordinators to keep handy while managing both legal and financial affairs.

YOUR LOVED ONE'S RIGHTS

While acting as proxy, you also will be an advocate to protect your loved one's rights. The key areas of interest are your loved one's rights as a patient, as an individual who is covered by health insurance, and as a person with a disability.

PATIENT BILL OF RIGHTS

Under federal and state law, everyone who is receiving medical care, including home care and residential treatment, is entitled to certain rights. The homecare agency is required by law to inform their clients of these rights (National Association for Home Care and Hospice [NAHC], n.d.). Ask to see this document in writing.

NAHC (n.d.) has developed its own bill of rights based on patient rights that are currently enforced. The following are some key elements of this document:

- Homecare agencies are required to provide information regarding all rights and responsibilities, appropriate information about the condition for the patient's informed consent to treatment, all policies, and charges, including those not covered by Medicare, Medicaid, or insurance.
- Healthcare providers are required to comply with advance directives according to state law.
- Patients have the right to refuse treatment, choose healthcare providers, and voice grievances without fear of retaliation or discrimination.
- Healthcare providers are required to notify patients within a reasonable amount of time regarding changes in the plan of care, transfer to another facility or healthcare provider, or termination of services.
- Healthcare providers are required to provide a reasonable continuity of care. The healthcare team works together to provide high-quality, cost-effective medical care and health management (American Academy of Family Physicians, n.d.).

PATIENT'S RIGHTS REINFORCED BY PRESIDENTIAL MEMORANDUM

On April 15, 2010, President Obama issued a memorandum to the secretary of the U.S. Department of Health and Human Services. In this memo, Obama requested that the department ensure that all hospitals receiving Medicare and Medicaid funding respect patients' wishes in regard to power of attorney for health care and advance directives. The memo also noted the patient's right to designate visitors. Although not official law, the memo reinforces existing laws and opens the door for new laws that protect patients and unrelated caregivers.

PATIENT'S RIGHT TO REVOKE THE ADVANCE DIRECTIVE

The patient can revoke the advance directive at any time, and if at any time the patient has the mental capacity and consciousness to make decisions, the healthcare team will refer to the patient rather than the proxy (Caritas Good Samaritan Medical Center, n.d.). This is important to keep in mind because many loved ones will take these documents as set in stone, and conflicts between family members may arise if the patient has the mental capacity to make a treatment choice that contradicts the advance directive.

For example, a loved one with a terminal degenerative disease decides in an advance directive that she wants to die at home. The proxy is visiting the patient and sees that she is in extreme pain and discomfort. The proxy asks the patient if she wants to go to the hospital. The loved one is unable to speak but nods vigorously. The loved one is clearly able to make the decision to go to the hospital, and despite a document that was made months ago, this current wish should be followed. However, if the loved one is aware enough to refuse medical treatment, this wish should be followed, even if medical treatment would ease the patient's suffering.

HEALTH INSURANCE REFORM LEGISLATION

On March 23, 2010, the president signed legislation that will begin to transform the health insurance system. However, this law is still in flux, as 14 states, including Florida, Texas, and Pennsylvania, are suing the federal government over the burden that the states will face to support this law (Wechsler, 2010).

Eighteen provisions are slated to become effective within a year of enactment. According to HealthReform.gov (n.d.), the key components that will most affect patients include the following:

- Health plans cannot discriminate against children based on a preexisting condition. (In 2014, this will apply to people of all ages.)
- Insurance companies are not allowed to drop people from coverage because of illness or injury.
- Children are allowed to remain under their parent's health insurance until their 26th birthday.
- An independent appeals process has been established with both external and internal channels so that people can appeal the decisions made by their insurance providers.
- Insurance companies will be held accountable for unreasonable rate hikes.

DISABILITY LEGISLATION

Although your loved one may not consider himself to have a disability, because he has a serious illness or injury, your loved one is entitled to certain rights under seven key federal laws (U.S. Department of Justice, 2005). Table 3 provides a brief description of these laws. Even if your loved one's condition is only temporary, it is important that he is treated fairly. Employers and public entities are required by law to comply; if they do not, you may consider seeking legal counsel to pursue the matter further.

Table 3. Rights for People With Disabilities Under Federal Laws	
Legislation	**Rights Provided**
Air Carrier Access Act	Domestic and foreign air carriers are not allowed to discriminate against people with physical or mental disabilities. Air carriers must provide boarding assistance and accessibility features.
	(Continued on next page)

Table 3. Rights for People With Disabilities Under Federal Laws *(Continued)*	
Legislation	**Rights Provided**
Americans With Disabilities Act	Employers, state and local governments, public accommodations and transportation, commercial businesses, and telecommunications are not allowed to discriminate against a person with a disability. People with disabilities have the right to equal opportunity, accessibility, and reasonable accommodation.
Civil Rights of Institutionalized Persons Act	The U.S. Attorney General has the authority to investigate institutions (including publicly operated nursing homes and psychiatric institutions) that are suspected of widespread deficiencies, including subjecting residents to harm, reprehensible conditions, and patterns of practice that deny residents' constitutional or federal rights.
Fair Housing Act	People with disabilities have the right to fair housing opportunities. Private, local, state, and federal owners are not allowed to discriminate against people with disabilities in renting or selling properties.
Individuals With Disabilities Education Act	Children with disabilities have the right to free public education that meets their needs.
Rehabilitation Act	Federal agencies and contractors and programs that receive federal financial assistance are not allowed to discriminate against people with disabilities in regard to participation and employment.
Telecommunications Act	Manufacturers of telecommunications equipment and service providers are required to ensure that equipment and services are accessible to people with disabilities.

Note. Based on information from U.S. Department of Justice, 2005.

YOUR RIGHTS AS CARE COORDINATOR

HEALTH INSURANCE PORTABILITY AND ACCOUNTABILITY ACT OF 1996

The Health Insurance Portability and Accountability Act of 1996 (HIPAA) is a federal law that protects patient information. HIPAA sets rules and limits on who can receive and view personal health data and gives individuals rights over their personal health information. It applies to all types of communication—written, electronic, and oral (U.S. Department of Health and Human Services [DHHS], n.d.). Healthcare providers, health insurance agencies, and their associated personnel must comply with patients' rights to receive a copy of all health records and make corrections to the health records and must notify patients about how and why their information was shared (DHHS, n.d.).

This legislation affects care coordinators in that providers and insurers are very careful about giving out information about the patient's condition to anyone other than the patient. Healthcare providers and insurers are allowed to share this information with family, friends, and other people that the patient identifies (DHHS, n.d.). To avoid delays and miscommunication, the patient should identify the family care coordinator as a person who is allowed to receive this information.

FAMILY AND MEDICAL LEAVE ACT OF 1993

In certain circumstances, employees have the right to take time away from their jobs to care for a family member in need. The Family and Medical Leave Act of 1993 (FMLA) allows employees to take up to 12 weeks off from their jobs for caregiving duties (U.S. Department of Labor [DOL], n.d.). Although employers are bound by law to grant leave, they are not required to pay a wage for it. However, during this time, health insurance must be continued without change, and the employee's job is protected. The employee may take leave under the FMLA in these three circumstances (DOL, n.d.):

- For the birth and care of a newborn or acquisition of a child for adoption or foster care
- For the care of an immediate family member (defined by DOL as a spouse, parent, or child)
- For the employee's own serious illness.

In October 2009, an amendment to FMLA went into effect called the National Defense Authorization Act for Fiscal Year 2010 (DOL Wage and Hour Division, 2010). This amendment provides additional protection for family members of injured and ill soldiers. The amendment applies to care coordinators of all active members of the Armed Forces, including the National Guard and the Reserves. It allows care coordinators up to 26 weeks of job-protected leave to help with medical treatment, therapy, and outpatient care for military personnel on active duty who are seriously ill, injured, or otherwise on the temporary disability retired list. To qualify, the care coordinator must be a spouse, son, daughter, parent, or next of kin (DOL Wage and Hour Division, 2010).

RIGHTS OF SAME-SEX PARTNERS AND UNRELATED CARE COORDINATORS

Although all care coordinators need to ensure that their loved ones' wishes about who is in charge of making decisions on their behalf, this is especially true for same-sex couples. In the United States, the legal rights of lesbian, gay, bisexual, and transgender (LGBT) couples vary from state to state. Currently, some states recognize LGBT marriages, but because of the unpredictable nature of politics, this right could be revoked with the next election. In addition, if a couple is considered legally married in one state but live in another that does not recognize the marriage, they are not guaranteed the same rights as other couples.

Some friends and neighbors who may be emotionally closer to the person in need than any biologic relative may face similar dilemmas. Unless the person states otherwise, when healthcare professionals look to someone to make medical decisions, they will seek out the biologic relatives first. Even if no relatives can be found, this can slow down the process and make the situation more stressful and difficult for everyone involved (Caritas Good Samaritan Medical Center, n.d.).

For same-sex partners, the first step is to investigate the local, state, and federal laws in the specific area where they reside. Some do not recognize marriage per se, but they call it something different, such as *domestic partnerships, civil unions,* and *reciprocal beneficiaries* (Family Caregiver Alliance, n.d.). The next step is to file the necessary paperwork to secure protection under existing laws. "Without legal protections in place, these relationships might not be legally recognized and could easily be questioned or contested by a biological family member" (Family Caregiver Alliance, n.d., para. 2).

Save all documentation, and place a copy of everything in a secure location, such as a safe-deposit box at a bank or a fireproof box at home. All documents should be carefully drafted and filed properly using the appropriate channels and protocols. Save proof of filing, including receipts and canceled checks, as well as dated instructions and protocols from the government agency where you are filing (these usually can be found on your state's Web site). The following documents should be prepared

as soon as you and your partner decide to enter into a committed relationship (Family Caregiver Alliance, n.d.):
• Will
• Living trust (or revocable trust)
• Durable powers of attorney for finances and health care.
In addition, if you and your partner have minor children, you will need documents that ensure that the children will stay with one of you in the event that the other is incapacitated or dies (Family Caregiver Alliance, n.d.).

For friends and neighbors who want to secure the same rights as family members, these four documents will also provide some protection of your loved one's wishes. Although biologic relatives can still go to court to challenge these documents, it will be difficult to dispute. As with same-sex partners, the earlier these decisions are made and legally documented, the better.

PLANNING FOR THE FUTURE

As a care coordinator, what happens if you become ill or injured, or if your loved one lives longer than you? As you assume responsibility for your loved one's affairs, this is a good time to review your own legal portfolio. This is especially important if you have a child with disabilities who will need lifelong care. Be sure to name a legal guardian and to make arrangements for care in the event that you are not able to provide it.

POINTS TO REMEMBER

• Enlist the help of legal counsel when taking over your loved one's affairs.

- While your loved one is still capable of making decisions, have a frank discussion about his values and wishes. In addition, organize all essential documents so that they are secure but accessible in case your loved one becomes incapacitated.
- Your loved one has rights as a patient, as a health insurance consumer, and as a person with a disability. Knowledge of these rights will help you ensure the best care and fairness for your loved one.
- Because HIPAA has specific rules about who is allowed to receive personal medical information, make sure your loved one identifies you as someone who can receive this information.
- If your loved one chooses you as her primary decision maker, visit a lawyer together to ensure that all the paperwork is in order and properly filed. Review these documents with your loved one's physician so that everyone is on the same page in regard to the meaning of medical terminology, treatments, and interventions.
- Open communication about your loved one's wishes and how those wishes may change depending on the situation with friends and family members will help prevent arguments and tensions later.
- If you are not the spouse or a close biologic relative to the person in need, your loved one must take the proper steps well in advance to ensure that your rights are protected and that the loved one's wishes are properly executed.
- Save and document everything.
- You are entitled to 12 weeks of unpaid leave (26 weeks for qualified care coordinators of military personnel) through FMLA.
- Many legal documents that give you permission to access and control your loved one's affairs must be filed by your loved

one. Having these documents prepared before illness will make the process a lot easier.

• Review your own legal portfolio, and include your loved one in your estate plans.

REFERENCES

American Academy of Family Physicians. (n.d.). Continuity of care, definition of. Retrieved from http://www.aafp.org/online/en/home/policy/policies/c/continuityofcaredefinition.html

American Bar Association Commission on Law and Aging. (n.d.). Guide for health care proxies. Retrieved from http://www.abanet.org/aging/toolkit/tool9.pdf

Caritas Good Samaritan Medical Center. (n.d.). Health care proxy: Frequently asked questions. Retrieved from http://www.caritasgoodsam.org/Documents/health%20care%20proxy%20faq.pdf

Family Caregiver Alliance. (n.d.). Legal issues for LGBT caregivers. Retrieved from http://www.caregiver.org/caregiver/jsp/content_node.jsp?nodeid=436&expandednodeid=387

HealthReform.gov. (n.d.). Key provisions that will take effect immediately. Retrieved from http://www.healthreform.gov/reports/keyprovisions.html

Iowa State Bar Association. (2004). What is a living trust? Retrieved from http://www.iowabar.org/Public%20Information%20Brochures.nsf/d7ff6dc91c517cdb862567ba00690c91/b597f0e72c1933f486256e280054c4a3!OpenDocument

National Association for Home Care and Hospice. (n.d.). What are my rights as a patient? Retrieved from http://www.nahc.org/consumer/rights.html

Obama, B. (2010, April 15). Presidential memorandum—hospital visitation [Memorandum]. Retrieved from http://www.whitehouse.gov/the-press-office/presidential-memorandum-hospital-visitation

Repa, B.K. (n.d.). Am I responsible for my father's nursing home bills? Retrieved from http://www.caring.com/questions/responsible-for-nursing-home-bills

Steinberg, B. (n.d.). Am I responsible for my parent's debt? Retrieved from http://www.caring.com/questions/responsible-for-nursing-home-bills

U.S. Department of Health and Human Services. (n.d.). Your health information is protected by federal law. Retrieved from http://www.hhs.gov/ocr/privacy/hipaa/understanding/consumers/index.html

U.S. Department of Justice. (2005, September). A guide to disability rights laws. Retrieved from http://www.ada.gov/cguide.htm

U.S. Department of Labor. (n.d.). The Family and Medical Leave Act. Retrieved from http://www.dol.gov/compliance/laws/comp-fmla.htm

U.S. Department of Labor Wage and Hour Division. (2010, February). Fact Sheet #28A: The Family and Medical Leave Act Military Family Leave Entitlements. Retrieved from http://www.dol.gov/whd/regs/compliance/whdfs28a.htm

Wechsler, P. (2010, March 23). States sue over overhaul that will bust state budgets (update 2). Retrieved from http://www.bloomberg.com/apps/news?pid=20601087&sid=ajwSWE6H1kHM

CHAPTER 5

HELP WANTED: FINANCIAL PLANNER

INTRODUCTION

A big stressor for caregivers and loved ones is how to pay for all of the expenses associated with long-term illness and disability. If the loved one was working prior to the injury or illness, the family will need to juggle its finances to compensate for the lack of income. Likewise, retired older adults may have fixed incomes and modest financial resources. Although the benefits for healthcare expenses may be limited, individuals with disabilities and long-term illnesses may qualify for programs that offer compensation for other expenses, such as food and transportation.

This chapter identifies some of the resources that are available to you and your loved one to ease the financial burden associated with disability and illness. Different types of insurance are described, as are the items needed to create an accurate snapshot of your loved one's financial situation. The chapter also discusses the government, nonprofit, and for-profit agencies that provide financial assistance.

ORGANIZATION

If your loved one in need is an independent adult, the first step is to have a discussion about his financial situation. As with legal matters, ideally this conversation will take place well before the loved one loses the ability to make financial decisions. Schedule a time to visit and have the discussion. Consider splitting the conversation into two meetings to discuss financial and legal matters if one such discussion would be too overwhelming for you or your loved one. Because this conversation may be a little tedious and frustrating, end the discussion by doing something relaxing together, such as going out to dinner or ordering in a favorite meal, watching a movie together, or taking a walk so that the visit ends on a positive note. Get the necessary paperwork together so you can manage your loved one's finances.

Financial Documents Checklist

Asset Documentation
- Tax records from at least the past five years
- Bank statements and account numbers from each institution, including checking, savings, and certificates of deposits
- Deeds and titles for property
- Investment documentation, including pension funds, 401(k) retirement accounts and individual retirement accounts (IRAs), stocks, and bonds
- Health savings account information

Debt Documentation
- Loans, including mortgages, home equity loans and lines of credit, reverse mortgages, liens, and vehicle and personal loans
- Credit card information, including account numbers and balances
- Utility bills, including account numbers and unpaid balances
- Unpaid taxes, including penalties and interest
- Any outstanding medical bills

(Continued on next page)

Financial Documents Checklist *(Continued)*

Insurance (for each policy)
- Effective dates
- Proof that the policy premium is paid and current
- Terms

Other Important Documents*
- Birth certificate
- Social Security card
- Military documentation
- Immigration or naturalization documents

*Government agencies and insurance companies may require these documents in order to process your loved one's claim for compensation.

INSURANCE

Insurance is a contract between you and an agency that says that as long as your premiums are paid, the agency will compensate you for any loss or damage that is covered by the contract terms. Many types of insurance exist to provide financial protection in a variety of circumstances. The most relevant types will be covered here. However, you should consult with a financial planner or insurance agent to determine what is available to you or to discuss liquidating policies that your loved one has.

SHORT-TERM DISABILITY INSURANCE

Short-term disability insurance is a benefit offered by some employers for financial protection in the event of an injury or illness that will require more time off than the amount of paid leave to which the employee is entitled. Usually, this benefit will pay 40%–65% of the employee's pretax salary for approximately three to six months or until the employee is cleared by a doctor to return to work, whichever comes first (Insure.com, 2010b). The insurance typically is an added benefit above and beyond other employer benefits and Social Security (Insure. com, 2010b).

LONG-TERM DISABILITY INSURANCE

Long-term disability insurance is another benefit employers may offer in case of illness or injury that exceeds the employee's paid leave. Usually, this benefit picks up when the short-term insurance coverage expires. Unfortunately, because this benefit is often optional and employees usually are responsible for the partial or total cost of the premiums, some opt to get only one type of insurance or none at all. If your loved one did not purchase short-term insurance but has long-term coverage, she may have to wait until enough time passes to collect compensation (check the details of the policy to confirm the criteria for compensation). Conversely, if your loved one chose short-term disability insurance but not long-term coverage, you will need to have a contingency plan in place once the benefit expires.

Depending on the policy, long-term disability insurance covers 50%–60% of the employee's salary (Insure.com, 2010a). The length of coverage varies from two years to until the employee turns 65 (Insure.com, 2010a). Similar to short-term coverage, if a person recovers and is able to return to work, a doctor's release can also terminate the benefit.

WORKERS' COMPENSATION

Workers' compensation is a type of insurance that all states (except Texas) require employers to have in the event of a workplace injury (AllBusiness.com, n.d.). The employer's insurance company usually pays for temporary or permanent disability wages, medical expenses related to the injury, and vocational rehabilitation if the worker can no longer perform the duties of the job because of the injury (FreeAdvice.com, 2008). A few restrictions apply, including if the worker sustained the injury while engaging in reckless behavior, while under the influence of drugs or alcohol, or while engaging in an illegal act, or if the employee intentionally caused the injury. In addition, if the worker was hurt while off duty, he may not be eligible for workers' compensation (AllBusiness.com, n.d.).

HEALTH INSURANCE

If your loved one has health insurance, this would be a good time to review all of the benefits and restrictions of the policy. Particular items to consider:

- Copayments—Are they all the same or do they vary among the types of practitioners?
- Does the policy have a deductible? A deductible is the amount of money the policy holder must pay in healthcare expenses before the coverage kicks in. Is the deductible for everything or just certain services?
- Are diagnostic services such as blood tests, sonograms, and x-rays covered?
- Are therapies such as physical therapy, mental health services, or chiropractic services covered? If so, does the policy include a limit, either in the number of visits or sessions or a dollar amount?
- Does the policy include a prescription drug benefit? Does it have a preference for generic drugs? Some policies have a drug formulary that lists the copayment for each type of drug by price category. Review this document so that you and your loved one can budget for prescription copayments.

- Does the policy include a benefit for durable medical equipment? Examples of durable medical equipment are crutches, braces, mobility equipment (wheelchairs, scooters), and prostheses. If this benefit is included, what type of equipment is covered? Does the policy have an annual limit or deductible for this provision?

As the care coordinator, you can provide a significant contribution by helping your loved one keep track of all claims (American Cancer Society, 2008). However, because of the Health Insurance Portability and Accountability Act of 1996 (HIPAA), the health insurance company will not be allowed to release any claim or medical information to you unless your loved one specifically signs a form giving you permission to receive this information. A complete explanation of HIPAA is found in Chapter 4.

AUTOMOBILE INSURANCE

If the disabling injury is the result of an automobile accident, sometimes automobile insurance will cover any related medical expenses. You will need to investigate your loved one's car insurance policy or the policy of the driver at fault to see if any coverage is available. An auto insurance agent will help you sort through these details.

LONG-TERM CARE INSURANCE

Long-term care insurance is a relatively new option that provides compensation in the event that an individual needs in-home healthcare services or to move into a long-term care facility. If your loved one has a policy, now is the time to review it and determine the length of coverage and whether it has a waiting period before reimbursement begins (for example, when the 90-day Medicare benefit for nursing home care expires). In addition, check the policy to see exactly what expenses it covers, such as specialized care or a private room.

SUPPLEMENTAL INSURANCE

This type of insurance is available through many agencies to provide an additional benefit as a complement to disability and health insurance. Some policies will provide payment for expenses such as food and transportation, whereas others will cover specific debts such as mortgages, home equity loans, automobile loans, and credit card payments if an individual is unable to work because of illness or injury.

LIFE INSURANCE

Some life insurance policies have cash value that can be tapped into when needed. Another way to access this money is to take out a loan against the policy at an interest rate that is often lower than a bank loan (Insure.com, 2008). The individual will not be required to return this money, but the beneficiaries' payout will be lower. Keep in mind that the most lucrative policies tend to be several years old, as cash value often grows much more slowly with life insurance policies than with other types of investments (Insure.com, 2008). It is important to review this option with a financial adviser, especially if you choose to tap into your own policy.

HEALTH SAVINGS ACCOUNTS

Health savings accounts are national savings programs created by Medicare that allow individuals to save for current and future medical expenses on a tax-free basis (U.S. Treasury Department, 2007). These accounts are used in conjunction with high-deductible health insurance plans. Both the employer and individual can make contributions to the account, and others may make deposits on the individual's behalf. No income limits exist for this program, but individuals who participate in this program have the following restrictions (U.S. Treasury Department, 2007):

- Participants cannot be enrolled in Medicare.
- Participants cannot be listed as a dependent on someone else's tax return.
- Participants cannot be covered by health insurance other than or in addition to the high-deductible plan.

HEALTHCARE AND DEPENDENT CARE FLEXIBLE SPENDING ACCOUNTS

Healthcare and dependent flexible spending accounts are pretax accounts sponsored by the federal government (FSA Feds, n.d.). Employers offer healthcare accounts to pay for out-of-pocket expenses not covered by other insurance. The dependent care option can be used to pay for child care and adult dependent care. Both types have a limited list of eligible expenses, and the dependent care account has specific requirements regarding paid caregivers and establishments providing care (for example, a day camp may be covered depending on the program, whereas music lessons would not be). A maximum of $5,000 can be saved in each type of account per year, and expenses cannot be claimed on an income tax return (FSA Feds, n.d.). Another catch is that all the money saved must be used within the calendar year, or it will be forfeited.

INCOME, ASSETS, DEBTS, AND EXPENSES

To develop an accurate idea of your loved one's financial situation, budget for the future, and determine available assets to pay for professional care, you need to take inventory of your loved one's current financial portfolio, including income, assets, debts, and expenses. Even if your loved one is no longer employed, income could be in the form of interest payments from a pension fund and Social Security retirement payments, stock dividends, and profit-sharing payouts.

Assets include any property of value, such as real estate and vehicles. Other assets include retirement savings, such as 401(k), individual retirement accounts, and pensions, traditional savings accounts, stocks, bonds, tax shelter accounts, money market accounts, and certificates of deposit. Find out where each account is held, as well as current balances and account numbers. Other resources of asset revenue include collections (such as antiques, coins, or art), furniture, appliances, electronics, musical instruments, and jewelry. This may be a good time to organize a yard sale or to consult an estate sale specialist to determine hidden value in the home.

Debts include all credit card balances, outstanding medical bills, vehicle loans, mortgages, home equity loans and lines of credit, unpaid tax balances, and other personal loans. Do not forget to total any outstanding balances for utility bills and other services.

Expenses include utilities, copayments for medication and doctor's visits, home and car maintenance, taxes, insurance premiums, food and personal care items, entertainment, and clothing. Other expenses include payments for services such as haircuts, lawn care, and home healthcare visits, and any regular donations that your loved one makes, such as to a religious organization.

Listing these items can help your loved one see on paper what money is available and determine priorities. Collect this information and keep it in a safe place where it can be quickly accessed, especially in the event that your loved one is unable to communicate. Reassess financial information periodically to keep the details current and relevant to your loved one's goals and situation. Enlist the help of a certified public accountant or a financial planner for more detailed tips and information.

FINANCIAL ASSISTANCE

Once the financial picture is complete, you can look to a variety of government agencies and other organizations to help with expenses. See Appendix 2 for a list of important Internet resources that can provide information regarding financial assistance. Many government agencies and nonprofit organizations offer high-demand programs that are managed by limited staff. It is important to be patient but persistent when applying for benefits. Keep all copies of all paperwork that you file, and take notes regarding phone conversations, including the names and titles of people you contacted. Programs may have waiting lists, so as soon as you identify a need and an agency that can provide help, contact the agency.

GOVERNMENT HELP

The federal government has a few health insurance programs; one such program is called Medicare. This program is for people who are age 65 or older, people who are younger than 65 with certain disabilities, and people who have kidney disease and require dialysis or a kidney transplant (Centers for Medicare and Medicaid Services, 2005). Part A coverage does not require a premium, and Part B has a monthly premium. Part C is insurance provided by Medicare-approved agencies (also called Medicare Advantage) that provides the same benefits as Parts A and B but offers provider flexibility (Medicare.gov, n.d.). A prescription drug benefit (Medicare Part D) is also available to those who qualify.

Medicaid is another program that offers financial assistance for health programs to people with low income, certain disabilities, and young children (Medical News Today, n.d.). Each state sets its own eligibility standards and covered services. The federal government also offers low-cost health insurance for children through the Children's Health Insurance Program, commonly referred to as CHIP. The application forms for government health insurance can be intimidating, but many community groups and hospitals offer help with navigating the process by providing seminars and individual consultation about these programs.

The Veterans Benefits Administration offers financial assistance for former military personnel and their families, including health insurance, compensation for service-related disabilities and sexual and emotional trauma, low-interest home loans, pensions, grants for assistive devices, and educational and vocational training assistance.

Social Security Disability and Supplemental Security Income programs are benefit programs supported by the federal government through the Social Security Tax. The programs provide monthly payments to people with disabilities, their spouses, and their children. Benefits are also available to children with disabilities based on payments their parents made into the program.

The U.S. Department of Housing and Urban Development (HUD) has several approved housing counseling agencies throughout the country that provide guidance on finding subsidized rent, purchasing a home, and avoiding foreclosure. Special programs are available for people with disabilities, low-income populations, and veterans.

Assistance for higher-education expenses is available from federal, state, and local governments through grants and low-interest loans for all people. People with disabilities and their children may also qualify for additional grants. In addition, children with special needs can qualify for preschool and other programs that are paid for by the local school district. Early intervention programs for children with intellectual, developmental, or physical disabilities are available to children as young as 18 months old and are designed to help these children to develop to their full potential, including integrating into a public school classroom with children their own age. School districts will also provide tutors to keep children with illnesses current with their class work when they are too ill to go to school; they also provide testing for learning disabilities. These services are usually free of charge. It is important to apply for these services as soon as possible because many have extensive waiting lists.

ASSISTANCE FROM OTHER AGENCIES

Many nonprofit and for-profit companies offer financial relief for older adults, people with disabilities, and families who are struggling financially. One place to start is to investigate relief options through your loved one's home utility providers, especially for natural gas and electricity. Utility companies offer budgeting plans to make the monthly payment smaller, and donations from other customers can help subsidize your loved one's bill. These programs are in place so that your loved one does not have to choose between having heat in the winter and paying for expensive medications.

Drug companies are another source of relief. If your loved one takes an expensive medication or has several prescriptions, investigate help from the drug maker. Some companies offer patient assistance programs that provide discounts and free medicine to people who are uninsured or underinsured or have a low income. These companies also work with doctors by providing a supply of free samples they can distribute to patients who meet the financial criteria. In addition, many organizations provide help with medication costs (see Appendix 2 for online resources).

Nonprofit disability- and disease-specific groups are another resource for financial help. Offerings vary from group to group and can include assistance with the costs of medical supplies and equipment, mobility equipment, prostheses and wigs, accommodations for the patient's family when traveling to distant hospitals for medical procedures, respite retreats, legal counsel, and much more. Chances are there is a group whose sole purpose is to help people like your loved one. If they do not provide money directly, most likely they can help you navigate the system to find financial resources. Some will even advocate on your loved one's behalf to secure these resources. Your loved one's social worker is a good resource for this type of information. In addition, the Internet provides a wealth of information and way to connect with organizations that serve people with your loved one's specific needs. The United Way (www.liveunited.org), a nonprofit network of more than 1,300 local organizations, is a good place to begin.

Philanthropic foundations, community groups, and religious organizations often have special programs for people in need. Some offer services, such as meal delivery programs and gatherings that offer low-cost or free meals. Others help with medical bills or fulfill specific unmet needs, such as building an access ramp or purchasing expensive equipment that would improve your loved one's quality of life. In addition, people from within the community may rally on your loved one's behalf to organize fund-raisers such as raffles, bake sales, dinners, or social events. Some foundations offer scholarships for students with a specific type of disability.

Many debt relief organizations are designed to negotiate lower payments and loan forgiveness for outstanding balances on medical bills, loans, and credit card debt. These services should be pursued with caution and under the advice of a financial expert or bankruptcy attorney. Although some reputable nonprofit agencies provide these services, others are not legitimate. It is important to note that debt relief agreements may provide only a temporary fix for financial problems and may hurt your loved one's or your credit rating.

A WORD ABOUT ACCEPTING FINANCIAL HELP

Some people are hesitant to accept help from the government or charitable organizations. Keep in mind that these programs were designed to be available for people in your family's situation. Read all the eligibility requirements, and if your loved one qualifies, accept the help. Many of these benefits and programs were started by people who were in your situation at one time and could not find the resources they needed. You can honor them by accepting help without shame and, when you are able to, show your gratitude through sending thank-you cards, writing letters to local newspapers, and volunteering for or donating to an organization that helped you.

BANKRUPTCY

Bankruptcy is a federal legal proceeding that helps individuals and businesses eliminate or repay debts under court protection (Nolo, n.d.). The most common types of bankruptcies are Chapter 7 and Chapter 13. Chapter 7 is a total liquidation of assets to pay for all or a portion of the debt, and the debt is forgiven. Chapter 13, on the other hand, establishes a payment plan to pay down debt over three to five years, usually followed by a discharge of the remaining debt (Ramsey, 2009). Bankruptcy is a last-resort solution, as this approach will devastate credit and make it difficult to get a loan.

Ramsey (2009) suggests avoiding bankruptcy completely, if possible. But if bankruptcy is absolutely necessary, you should contact an experienced bankruptcy attorney. Contacting an experienced financial planner is paramount, especially if you are considering using your own income or assets to fund care for someone other than an immediate relative, as this can cause devastating financial consequences.

POINTS TO REMEMBER

- An assessment of your loved one's finances will help you identify the resources available to pay for healthcare expenses.
- Your loved one may have many types of insurance that will cover some of these expenses.

- Long-term care insurance, flexible spending accounts, and health savings accounts are options that can cover expenses that traditional health insurance does not.
- Many government and nonprofit agencies offer relief from the financial burdens of disability and chronic illness.
- Financial help is available for a reason. If you or your loved one meet the qualifications, take it, and then pay it forward when you are able.

REFERENCES

AllBusiness.com. (n.d.). Understanding workers' compensation. Retrieved from http://www.allbusiness.com/human-resources/benefits-insurance-workers-compensation/1319-1.html

American Cancer Society. (2008). *Cancer caregiving A to Z*. Washington, DC: Author.

Centers for Medicare and Medicaid Services. (2005). Medicare program general information. Retrieved from http://www.cms.hhs.gov/Medicare GenInfo

FreeAdvice.com. (2008, September). Employment labor law: What benefits are typically available under workers' compensation? Retrieved from http://employment-law.freeadvice.com/employment-law/benefits_compensation.htm

FSA Feds (n.d.). Health care and dependent care accounts: Summary of benefits with frequently asked questions. Retrieved from https://www.fsafeds.com/fsafeds/SummaryOfBenefits.asp#WhatIsFSA

Insure.com. (2008, May). Cash value in life insurance: What is it worth to you? Retrieved from http://www.insure.com/articles/lifeinsurance/cash-value.html

Insure.com. (2010a, January). The basics of long-term disability insurance. Retrieved from http://www.insure.com/articles/disabilityinsurance/long-term-disability.html

Insure.com. (2010b, January). The basics of short-term disability insurance. Retrieved from http://www.insure.com/articles/disabilityinsurance/short-term-disability.html

MedicalNewsToday. (n.d.). What is Medicare/Medicaid? Retrieved from http://www.medicalnewstoday.com/info/medicare-medicaid/whatismedicaid.php

Medicare.gov. (n.d.). Medicare Advantage (Part C). Retrieved from http://
www.medicare.gov/navigation/medicare-basics/medicare-benefits/
part-c.aspx

Nolo. (n.d.). What is bankruptcy? Retrieved from http://www.nolo.com/
legal-encyclopedia/article-29829.html

Ramsey, D. (2009, August 9). The truth about bankruptcy. Retrieved from
http://www.daveramsey.com/article/the-truth-about-bankruptcy

U.S. Treasury Department. (2007, July 22). All about HSAs. Retrieved from
http://www.ustreas.gov/offices/public-affairs/hsa/pdf/all-about-HSAs
_072208.pdf

CHAPTER 6

HELP WANTED: FAMILY COUNSELOR

INTRODUCTION

As the care coordinator for your loved one, you will face many emotional challenges. Your loved one will rely on you for not only physical support but also emotional and spiritual support. You may have to problem solve and mediate conflicts between family members. This chapter is about some of the social and emotional hurdles of caregiving.

JUST LISTEN

A big part of your job in providing emotional support for your loved one and other family members who are dealing with your loved one's illness or disability will be to just listen. You do not need to have all the answers or provide some insightful or witty comment; you just have to be there with ears and heart open. Actually, this may not be as easy as it sounds, especially in a loud and hectic world. Here are some pointers to be a more effective listener.

PRESENCE

Presence does not mean that you are just physically in the room with a person (or on the telephone, whatever the case may be). It means that your attention is focused on the person and on the moment. The past does not matter, nor does the future: just right here, right now.

DETACHMENT

Detachment is a good skill to learn because you have your own concerns, distress, emotional pain, and fear. Detachment from a situation will keep your mind from reeling as a doctor tells you and your loved one about a complex or devastating diagnosis. It is a skill that takes practice. You must first acknowledge that it is a stressful, sad, or worrisome situation. Then, focus on the doctor's or your loved one's words and say to yourself, "I'm not going to be upset about this now. Right now, I need to focus on getting all the information. Later, I will sit down alone and decide what this all means." Then you become an observer to the situation. Watch and listen closely without judgment, and document everything as much as you can by taking notes.

The trick is to actually keep that appointment with yourself so that your emotional needs are met. Temporary detachment is an effective tool because you can listen and gain information without your emotions clouding your attention. You can be supportive of your loved one instead of being distracted by your own fears. But, again, it is only a temporary fix. You must also take time for yourself emotionally and allow your loved one to support you as well.

LISTENING TYPES

Passive listening is when a person just sits and listens. The person does not offer any feedback and just takes in what the speaker has to say. This is best done without distraction so that the listener can be engaged and attentive (Negotiation Experts, n.d.; Paul & Paul, 2002).

Active listening is "a person's willingness and ability to hear and understand" (Hoppe, 2006, p. 12). Effective active listening can be accomplished with the following (Hoppe, 2006):

- Confirming that you are paying attention. Repeat what your loved one has just said, ask questions, or encourage your loved one to expand on a thought or to provide examples. Ask how you can help to make your loved one feel better or improve her situation.

- Sharing your view of the situation. You can provide your personal experiences and feelings so that your loved one can understand how you are feeling. It may be difficult, but open communication will help your relationship and you can lean on each other for support during a difficult time. Sharing your feelings and taking comfort from your loved one will empower and make her feel useful, needed, and loved.

- Choosing a quiet place that is free from distractions. This goes back to the presence idea. It is difficult to have a meaningful conversation with the television on or while you are doing something else that has your attention divided.

- Monitoring emotions. Choose a time when both of you are calm. It is difficult to listen when you are upset. Storming off is not the best approach; however, you can take a deep breath and say, "OK, we're both upset. Let's talk about it later this evening after we've had a chance to think about things and calm down."

CHOOSE YOUR WORDS WISELY

The companion to listening is speaking, and words can sting even in the best relationships under the best circumstances. However, in the case of a traumatic and burdensome health crisis, words can weigh much more heavily than they usually do on all family members. To effectively communicate with your loved ones under these sometimes tense circumstances, choose your words carefully, delicately, and compassionately. The adage "think before you speak" has never been truer than when describing the care coordinator/loved one relationship. Of course, all people lose their temper and say things they do not mean from time to time, but if you have a few key phrases on hand, the conversation will be less likely to take a negative turn (see Table 4). A good rule is to treat your family with the same courtesy and respect as you would a stranger.

Table 4. Effective Communication Phrases	
Instead Of	**Say**
Oh, you shouldn't feel that way!	I'm surprised to hear you say that. Why do you feel that way?
I don't get you sometimes.	What am I missing here? Please explain.
Control yourself. Calm down.	I see that you're upset right now. It's okay to cry. Let's find somewhere to talk about this in private. I'll be ready to listen when you're ready to talk about it.

(Continued on next page)

Table 4. Effective Communication Phrases *(Continued)*	
Instead Of	**Say**
How dare you accuse me . . .	I'm curious why you would think that I would . . .
We can do this the easy way or the hard way.	Which would you prefer?
Note. Based on information from Kreamer, 2010; Lenski, 2008; Whitehead, 2009; Zander, 2009.	

TAKE A WALK IN THEIR SHOES

In this emotionally charged time, it is easy to fall back into habits of taking offense at things people say, becoming annoyed by unusual or insensitive behavior, or judging people harshly. "Just" is an easy word to use at this time: He's just old. She's just acting like a rebellious teenager. He's just senile. You're just doing that to bug me. They're just greedy. Everyone is just ignoring me!

Whenever these "just" statements come to mind, that is a cue for you to dig a little deeper. Understanding other people's motivation or causes for their behavior will help you avoid anger and negative feelings toward people. Become curious. Ask your loved ones questions about how they are feeling and why they say what they say. Talk to a doctor, nurse, or social worker who has experience with your loved one's illness or injury about any strange behavior or an unusually short temper.

- Is your loved one staying up all night with the lights on and the television loud because she's *just* insensitive, or is her pain keeping her up at night? Could it be the medication she's taking? Is she worried about something?

- Did your loved one stop eating because he's *just* given up, or is this a natural part of the disease process or treatment?
- Is your loved one really *just* ignoring you, or is she having trouble hearing you?
- Are family members *just* being nosy and grim when they offer to make funeral arrangements, or are they sincerely trying to be helpful?

Investigating people's motivations may leave you feeling disappointed, but chances are, most people's intentions are good and there is a reasonable explanation behind distressing behavior and comments. This will also allow you to relate to other people a little better, to understand their fears and unique perspective on the situation, and to promote understanding and communication among all who are close to your loved one.

EMOTIONAL CHALLENGES BY RELATIONSHIP TYPE

Each relationship is different, and when relationships are challenged by a major illness, other issues arise. Here are a few things to expect when illness or disability happens, organized by relationship type.

PARENT

As mentioned in the introduction, the age at which a child will have to step in and take care of a parent is becoming younger and younger. It may seem like just yesterday you were moving out and establishing your own life when your parent faces a devastating illness, and from your parent's perspective, it may seem like just yesterday when he or she was changing your diapers or teaching you how to ride a bicycle. Your parent may be uncomfortable with the role reversal because he or she may still view you as a child rather than a competent adult. Old caregiving habits are hard to break.

You can make this reversal easier by reassuring your parent that it is a natural part of life for the child to take a turn at caring for the parent. Allow your parent to be a parent; illness does not take that privilege away entirely. Continue to ask for advice, and as long as your parent is physically able, allow him to do things for you, such as prepare your favorite meal. Include the person in family activities by visiting on holidays and sharing photos or videos of special occasions or events that he or she may not have been well enough to attend.

CHILD

When your child is ill, it can be devastating. In this situation, it is very tempting to be overprotective. Allowing your child to be a kid as much as possible will help to keep her on track for emotional, social, and mental development. When your child is a bit older, such as a teenager or young adult, you may be tempted to revert back to the days when you had more control over your child's life. Remember to respect your adult child's privacy and boundaries. Allow your teen to find comfort in his friends by encouraging frequent visits, and if your child is well enough, allow him to attend major school functions such as dances or sporting events. Even if the visits are brief or if the child can only stay at an event for 20 minutes before feeling tired, this will allow him to feel connected with his friends and peers.

If you have other children, it is often a delicate balance to give all the children equal attention, especially when a child is ill or has special needs. You can make a special effort to do things together as a family and to have one-on-one time with each child. Allow all children to be involved in family chores, decisions (choosing dinner or the movie, for example), and activities to a level based on their abilities and age.

Take advantage of some of the respite opportunities mentioned in Chapter 2. These will allow the family to create bonds with each other and for children to foster independence.

SIBLING

When your brother or sister is the loved one in need, sometimes your role as caregiver can be a peripheral one unless spouses and children are unable to fulfill this role. Younger siblings who are taking care of older ones may face the same role-reversal challenges as they would with a parent.

If you are a peripheral caregiver, you have the important task of acting as support for your sibling's spouse and children. You may have feelings of helplessness, but you can empower yourself by offering respite care and help with some of the chores of caregiving, such as grocery shopping, laundry, and running errands. You can make yourself available to your sibling's family by offering to listen or to help with medical decisions. When you offer love and kindness to your sibling's family, you will honor your sibling just as much as if you were taking care of him directly.

SPOUSE OR SIGNIFICANT OTHER

Randy Pausch, the late professor who wrote *The Last Lecture* about dealing with terminal cancer, described his relationship with his wife during his illness: "For starters, the best caregiving advice we've ever heard comes from flight attendants: 'Put on your own oxygen mask before assisting others'" (Pausch & Zaslow, 2008, p. 200). He and his wife attended counseling and worked together on daily tasks and leaned on each other for support. Serious illness or disability will probably be the biggest challenge in your relationship; take care of yourselves as individuals and take care of each other.

Pausch made a special effort to make memories with his three young children before he died. He had special outings with them and took a lot of photographs so they would remember him (Pausch & Zaslow, 2008). As a care coordinator for a spouse or partner, you can help your loved one to remain a special part of your children's or grandchildren's lives by making these kinds of memories.

Probably the furthest thing from your mind right now is your personal relationship with your partner. However, just because your partner is sick or injured does not mean that your relationship becomes a strictly nurse/patient professional relationship. Many couples lose intimacy in the day-to-day tasks of meeting the injured or ill partner's needs. This part of your relationship might seem dormant, but it is still there. Part of your partner's healing and recovery process will be to explore what it means to be a sexual being after a traumatic illness or injury (Katz, 2009, 2010).

At first, hugging and holding hands may be all that your loved one will be able to do, but as your partner becomes stronger, reintroduce yourselves to each other slowly and openly (Katz, 2009, 2010). Physical closeness will help to comfort both you and your loved one during this difficult time. Schedule regular "grown-up alone time" with no children, doctors, visitors, or interruptions (Katz, 2009, 2010). Privacy can be at a premium at this time, but it is important for your relationship.

ADDRESSING YOUR FEELINGS

Detachment is a wonderful thing, but it can only work for so long. Eventually, you will have to confront your own feelings about a situation. Caregiving brings with it some powerful and positive emotions: love, accomplishment, respect, connection, empowerment, and joy. However, caregivers face the negative emotions as well: guilt, anger, fear, sadness, exhaustion, feeling overwhelmed, disheartened, helplessness, loss (Berman, 2006).

Knowledge is a powerful antidote to feelings of helplessness and fear. Learn more about your loved one's disease and how to navigate the healthcare system. Ask for help, and attend a support group specific to your loved one's condition or for caregivers. This also would be a good time to rally the emotional troops of your friends, family, and spiritual leaders. You may be surprised by who you can count on when you ask for support, but the key is to ask.

The important thing is that negative emotions are natural and we all have bad days—cut yourself some slack for being angry or frustrated with your loved one. The Better Health Channel (1999) offers some general advice on dealing with negative emotions:

- Do not allow the same negative thoughts to echo in your head over and over again. Do not hold onto things that have happened in the past. Let go of grudges. Forgive. Focus on the present and the future.
- Engage in positive activities that will make you feel good about yourself. Allow time for your hobbies, exercise, and fun activities with both your loved one and other people. Make an appointment with yourself to watch your favor-

ite television show, go to a sporting event, have coffee or a night out with friends, or just spend some time alone—and stick to it.

- Learn about yourself and your loved one. Notice what triggers negative emotions so that you can be prepared to deal with them or defuse them by changing negative patterns that you and your loved one have established.

LONG-DISTANCE CAREGIVING

People who live far away from loved ones have a set of emotional challenges different from those who live nearby (Murphy, n.d.). You may feel guilty for not being there every day for the loved one in need, worry that he or she is not receiving proper care, or have feelings of disconnection and frustration for delays in receiving information (Murphy, n.d.).

Approximately 15% of caregivers are in the challenging position of caring for a person who lives an hour or more away (MetLife & National Alliance for Caregiving, 2005). Organization and communication are paramount in caring for a loved one from a distance. Forming a support network of other family members, neighbors, and healthcare professionals will help make your job easier. Enlisting the help of a professional care manager is a good alternative if no one is willing or able to deal with immediate responsibilities (MetLife & National Alliance for Caregiving, 2005). Professional care managers and social workers are good resources because they are neutral parties who may avert or help resolve family disputes regarding your loved one's care. Your loved one's physician, local hospital, or the local Department of Welfare office can put you in touch with one of these professionals.

Maintaining contact is important for both your peace of mind and your loved one's spirit. Send letters and cards, e-mail, call often, and mail care packages with photos, gifts, funny local stories or cartoons from the newspaper, and special treats. If you have children, nothing brightens a room like little ones' works of art. Regular contact will make the time between visits seem shorter for both of you.

VETERANS' SPECIAL NEEDS

As of December 31, 2009, 3.1 million veterans were receiving Veterans Administration disability compensation (U.S. Department of Veterans Affairs, 2010). Veterans of military service have a unique set of challenges in regard to disability and illness related to active duty. In addition to the physical trauma, many veterans who were on active duty during wartime may suffer from post-traumatic stress disorder (PTSD), a complex psychological disorder, as a response to traumatic experiences of war (James, 2010). PTSD can be so severe that the veteran is unable to work and interact socially.

Female veterans have the challenge of navigating a veterans' healthcare system that is designed for men (James, 2010). In addition, many problems, especially psychological and emotional problems, may go undiagnosed because women are trained that complaining is a sign of weakness. Women in the military may be victims of sexual assault that goes unreported (James, 2010). Caregivers have the role in these situations to observe veterans carefully for emotional distress and to encourage them to seek proper medical attention and counseling.

END-OF-LIFE CONCERNS

In the previous chapters, we discussed some of the legal and financial aspects that people must deal with when their loved ones are seriously ill and perhaps at the end of life: wills, guardianship of minor children, and power of attorney for finances. Of course, many emotions are involved with watching a loved one face the end of life.

PLANNING FOR THE END

If able, your loved one may want to be involved in planning funeral arrangements. If your loved one is an older adult, he may have already planned for this to an extent. Many funeral homes and cemeteries offer pre-need packages that allow a person to choose the casket, burial plot, and headstone, as well as other details regarding the funeral and burial.

Discussing funeral and burial arrangements with your loved one and other family members will give your loved one a sense of control and will give you peace of mind that your loved one's wishes have been honored. Your loved one may want to choose a particular outfit, the funeral home, whether to have a closed- or open-casket ceremony, or whether the service will be religious or secular. In regard to the actual burial, your loved one may prefer a space in a mausoleum rather than a plot in the ground with a headstone, or may want to forgo all that and be cremated. Your loved one can also provide input about people who might speak at the funeral and whether to ask people to donate to an organization in lieu of flowers. This discussion should also include exploring your loved one's priorities and beliefs about spirituality, religion, organ donation, and your loved one's legacy.

THE EMOTIONS OF LOSS

Grief is a very powerful swirl of emotions including sadness, anger, fear, and even relief. If your loved one has suffered a long illness, you may have experienced *anticipatory grief*, meaning that you have been grieving the loss of your loved one throughout your loved one's illness, perhaps even when you first learned of the diagnosis (Family Caregiver Alliance, 1996). You may have feelings of guilt or dread because of the burden of caring for your loved one or the difficulty of seeing your loved one in pain (Family Caregiver Alliance, 1996). All of these are natural emotions that people experience.

The length of time that people experience mourning and grief varies (Family Caregiver Alliance, 1996). However, if you feel unusually overcome by negative emotions and have trouble returning to your regular activities, talk to a professional about it. Spiritual leaders, mental health professionals, and even your primary care doctor can suggest ways to cope with grief. Support groups are also a helpful way to deal with loss. GriefShare's online search page (www.griefshare.org/find agroup) allows you to search for support groups by location. In addition, the Children's Grief Education Association (http://childgrief.org/childgrief.htm) is an online resource that provides information on how to help a child through feelings of loss and grief.

POINTS TO REMEMBER

- Listen!
- Learn the skill of detachment so that you avoid becoming emotional during critical times, such as when you need to hear medical information.

- However, be sure to address your feelings.
- Choose your words carefully and compassionately.
- Walk in other people's shoes.
- Negative emotions are normal, but don't allow them to control you.
- Each relationship has special challenges when a loved one becomes ill.
- Help your loved one create special memories with the family despite the illness.
- Build a team and enlist the help of a care manager or a social worker when caregiving long distance.
- Veterans have special emotional needs. Watch for signs of emotional and psychological distress, and seek counseling.
- Involving your loved one in the end-of-life process can be comforting for both of you.
- Feelings of grief are natural, and resources are available to help you and your children recover from loss.

REFERENCES

Berman, C. (2006). *Caring for yourself while caring for your aging parents: How to help, how to survive* (3rd ed.). New York, NY: Owl Books.

Better Health Channel. (1999). Negative emotions—coping tips. Retrieved from http://www.betterhealth.vic.gov.au/bhcv2/bharticles.nsf/pages/Negative_emotions_coping_tips

Family Caregiver Alliance. (1996, December). Grief and loss. Retrieved from http://www.caregiver.org/caregiver/jsp/content_node.jsp?nodeid=404

Hoppe, M.H. (2006). *Active listening: Improve your ability to listen and lead.* Greensboro, NC: Center for Creative Leadership.

James, S.D. (2010, March 2). Traumatized female vets face uphill battle. Retrieved from http://abcnews.go.com.print?id=9979866

Katz, A. (2009). *Woman cancer sex.* Pittsburgh, PA: Hygeia Media.

Katz, A. (2010). *Man cancer sex.* Pittsburgh, PA: Hygeia Media.

Kreamer, P. (2010, April). *Kreamer connection*. Pittsburgh, PA: Kreamer Connect Inc.

Lenski, T. (2008). 7 phrases you can't say in conflict resolution. Retrieved from http://conflictzen.com/7-phrases-you-cant-say-in-conflict-resolution

MetLife & National Alliance for Caregiving. (2005). SinceYouCare®: Long-distance caregiving. Retrieved from http://www.longdistancecaregiving.com/Long_Distance_Caregiving_Subject.pdf

Murphy, C. (n.d.). Long distance caregiver—coping with emotions. Retrieved from http://www.caregiver.com/channels/long_distance/articles/Care ForTheCaregiver/long_distance_caregiver.htm

Negotiation Experts. (n.d.). Acquiring good negotiating listening skills. Retrieved from http://www.negotiations.com/articles/listening-skills

Paul, J., & Paul, M. (2002). *Do I have to give up me to be loved by you?* (2nd ed.). Center City, MN: Hazelden.

Pausch, R., & Zaslow, J. (2008). *The last lecture*. New York, NY: Hyperion.

U.S. Department of Veterans Affairs. (2010, February). VA benefits and health care utilization. Retrieved from http://www1.va.gov/VETDATA/Pocket-card/4X6_winter10_sharepoint.pdf

Whitehead, S. (2009, December). Five phrases to embrace and five to avoid when talking to patients. Retrieved from http://www.emsresponder.com/print/EMS-Magazine/The-Power-of-Words/1$11261

Zander, K. (2009, August). Use these phrases to avoid conflict with patients, families, colleagues. *Patient Access Weekly Advisor*. Retrieved from http://www.hcpro.com/REV-237930-5354/Use-these-phrases-to-avoid-conflict-with-patients-families-colleagues.html

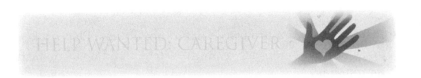

APPENDIX 1

CAREGIVER AND PATIENT SAFETY TIPS

BASIC SAFETY TIPS

- Learn cardiopulmonary resuscitation (CPR) and the Heimlich maneuver. Many hospitals, colleges, and YMCA centers offer classes for a nominal fee. Ask your loved one's physician if any modifications are needed related to your loved one's condition.
- Assemble a basic first aid kit or purchase a prefilled kit for the home. Add items specific to your family's needs, such as an EpiPen® (Dey Pharmaceuticals) for people with serious food or insect-bite allergies. Check expiration dates on contents every six months and replace outdated items.

HOME SAFETY

- Have a professional inspect the furnace, air conditioning unit, and electric service.
- Install smoke and carbon monoxide detectors. Check batteries frequently.

- Invest in a few multipurpose fire extinguishers. Place in key areas of the home, such as in the kitchen and near medical equipment.
- Use extra care in homes with oxygen tanks. Place signs on doors to warn visitors. Keep the oxygen tank away from open flame, such as fireplaces, stoves, and portable heaters. Make the home a no-smoking zone.
- Consider a home security system that includes a personal safety monitor. If your loved one becomes ill or injured when no one else is at home, the individual will be able to contact help by pushing a button on a bracelet or pendant.
- Properly discard medical waste. Contact your waste management provider for rules and instructions.
- Prevent accidental scalding by using a thermometer in the bath or shower and by setting the hot water tank to 120°F or lower (Visovsky et al., 2009).
- Prevent falls by rearranging furniture to provide a clear path, securing electrical cords, removing throw rugs and other tripping hazards, and rearranging shelves so that commonly used items are easily accessible without a stepladder (Visovsky et al., 2009).

MEDICATION

- Store all medications in a central location out of reach of children and pets.
- Keep a list of all medications, supplements, and herbal remedies, including the dosage amount and schedule. Make several copies and provide this information to all health providers and the pharmacist. Place the list with the medications where it can be easily seen. Include instructions on where

to find special medications that are separate from the main group, such as those that need to be refrigerated. Update this list as treatment regimens change.

- Follow all instructions exactly.
- Invest in a plastic pill organizer that includes slots for the day of the week as well as morning and evening. Help your loved one to fill each section carefully.
- Do not try to "stretch" medication by reducing doses or cutting pills in half. If you or your loved one need help paying for medications, tell the physician. Some may have free samples, and programs are available to help with medication costs.
- If your loved one's health insurance has limits on how often medications can be refilled or if you are using a mail-order service, be sure to keep track of when medications will need to be refilled so that your loved one doesn't run out before the next refill arrives.
- Review items in the medicine cabinet every six months and discard all medications, treatments, and supplements that have reached their expiration dates.
- If you help your loved one administer medications by injection, use needles only once and report any needlesticks to your physician.
- Keep the number of your local poison control center handy in case of accidental overdose. The national hotline is 800-222-1222.

RECOGNIZE AN EMERGENCY

Ask the doctor or nurse about emergency situations that could occur related to your loved one's specific condition, as well as what situations warrant a call to the doctor's office (for example, when a fever reaches a certain temperature or lasts a certain amount of time) and when to call emergency services. Regardless of your loved one's condition, if any of the following occur, call 911 immediately (Lake-Sumter Emergency Medical Services, n.d.):

- Difficulty breathing
- Swelling of the tongue, face, or throat
- Difficulty swallowing
- Choking
- Drowning
- Chest pain
- Slurred speech, paralysis on one side of the body, or severe headache
- Fainting, loss of consciousness, or unresponsiveness
- Seizures or convulsions
- Bleeding: Coughing up or vomiting blood, severe vaginal hemorrhage, or bleeding that won't stop
- Drug overdose or poisoning
- Overexposure to the elements, such as hypothermia (abnormally low body temperature) or suspected heat exhaustion or heat stroke.

CAREGIVER SAFETY

- Wear gloves when handling bed linens, incontinence protection (diapers, disposable bed pads), clothing, and other items soiled by bodily fluids (blood, vomit, urine). Take the same care as hospital personnel. Ask homecare personnel for advice and proper clean-up techniques.

- Take care to prevent back injury and falls when lifting and moving a patient. Use assistance devices and mobility aids, lift with the legs, and do not twist.
- Be sure to get adequate rest.
- Do not drive when overly tired.
- Protect your own health with proper nutrition and regular physician checkups.
- Make sure that all of your immunizations are current, especially if you are providing direct care to the patient. Your doctor can advise about whether it is necessary to receive vaccines for influenza, pneumonia, H1N1 (swine flu), or tetanus, as well as any other appropriate vaccines.

REFERENCES

Lake-Sumter Emergency Medical Services. (n.d.). When to call 911: What are some examples? Retrieved from http://www.whentocall911.com/whatexamples.htm

Visovsky, C., Collins, M.L., Hart, C., Abbott, L.I., & Aschenbrenner, J.A. (2009). ONS PEP resource: Peripheral neuropathy. In L.H. Eaton & J.M. Tipton (Eds.), *Putting evidence into practice: Improving oncology patient outcomes* (pp. 243–252). Pittsburgh, PA: Oncology Nursing Society.

APPENDIX 2
INTERNET RESOURCES

CAREGIVER RESOURCES

- Caregiver Resource Network: www.caregiverresource.net
- Family Caregiver Alliance: www.caregiver.org
- National Caregivers Library: www.caregiverslibrary.org
- Today's Caregiver: www.caregiver.com

KEY GOVERNMENT AGENCIES

- Administration for Children and Families: www.acf.hhs.gov
- Administration on Aging: www.aoa.gov
- Administration on Developmental Disabilities: www.acf.hhs .gov/programs/add
- Centers for Medicare and Medicaid Services: www.cms.hhs .gov
- Department of Housing and Urban Development: http://portal .hud.gov/portal/page/portal/HUD
- Department of Veterans Affairs: www.va.gov

- Healthcare reform information: www.healthreform.gov
- Medicare information: www.medicare.gov
- National Clearinghouse for Long-Term Care Information: www.longtermcare.gov/LTC/Main_Site/index.aspx
- Social Security Administration (includes Supplemental Security Income program): www.ssa.gov
- State Web sites (each state site has contact information for state agencies and state and federal legislature): www.usa.gov/Agencies/State_and_Territories.shtml

PRESCRIPTION AND COPAYMENT ASSISTANCE PROGRAMS

- HealthWell Foundation: www.healthwellfoundation.org
- National Alliance on Mental Illness Patient Prescription Drug Assistance Programs: http://www.nami.org/Content/ContentGroups/Helpline1/Prescription_Drug_Patient_Assistance_Programs.htm
- NeedyMeds: www.needymeds.org
- Partnership for Prescription Assistance: www.pparx.org/en
- Patient Advocate Foundation Co-Pay Relief Program: www.copays.org
- RxAssist directory of patient assistance programs: www.rxassist.org

OTHER SITES OF INTEREST

- American Association of People With Disabilities: www.aapd.com

- Independent Living Research Utilization National Directory of Centers for Independent Living: www.ilru.org/html/publications/directory/index.html
- National Council on Independent Living: www.ncil.org
- National Organization on Disability: www.nod.org